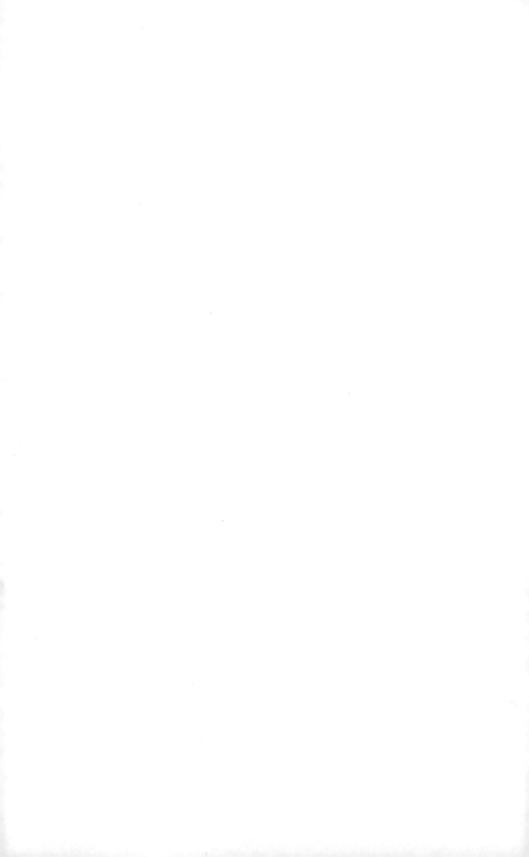

Cardiovascular Disease

METHODS IN MOLECULAR MEDICINE™

John M. Walker, SERIES EDITOR

METHODS IN MOLECULAR MEDICINE™

Cardiovascular Disease

Methods and Protocols
Volume 1: Genetics

Edited by

Qing K. Wang, PhD, MBA

Department of Molecular Medicine
Cleveland Clinic Lerner College of Medicine
Case Western Reserve University, Cleveland, OH

HUMANA PRESS ✳ TOTOWA, NEW JERSEY

© 2006 Humana Press Inc.
999 Riverview Drive, Suite 208
Totowa, New Jersey 07512

www.humanapress.com

This publication is printed on acid-free paper. ∞
ANSI Z39.48-1984 (American Standards Institute)
Permanence of Paper for Printed Library Materials.

Production Editor: Jennifer Hackworth

Cover illustration: Figure 2 from Volume 2, Chapter 13, "Methods for Isolation of Endothelial and Smooth Muscle Cells and In Vitro Proliferation Assays" by Ganapati H. Mahabeleshwar, Payaningal R. Somanath, and Tatiana V. Byzova

Cover design by Patricia F. Cleary

For additional copies, pricing for bulk purchases, and/or information about other Humana titles, contact Humana at the above address or at any of the following numbers: Tel.: 973-256-1699; Fax: 973-256-8341; E-mail: orders@humanapr.com; or visit our Website: www.humanapress.com

Printed in the United States of America. 10 9 8 7 6 5 4 3 2 1
1-59745-159-2 (e-book)

Library of Congress Cataloging in Publication Data
   Cardiovascular disease : methods and protocols / edited by Qing
Wang.
     v. ; cm. -- (Methods in molecular medicine ; 128-129)
   Includes bibliographical references and index.
   Contents: v. 1. Genetics -- v. 2. Molecular medicine.
   ISBN 1-58829-572-9 (v. 1 : alk. paper) -- ISBN 1-58829-892-2 (v. 2 :
alk. paper)
   1. Cardiovascular system--Diseases--Genetic aspects--Laboratory
manuals. I. Wang, Qing, 1965- . II. Series.
   [DNLM: 1. Cardiovascular Diseases--genetics--Laboratory Manuals.
2. Cardiovascular Diseases--physiopathology--Laboratory Manuals.
3. Molecular Biology--methods--Laboratory Manuals.   WG 25 C2678
2006]
   RC687.C37 2006
   616.1'042--dc22   2006000450

Preface

Cardiovascular disease is the leading cause of death in developed countries, but is quickly becoming an epidemic in such well-populated countries as China, India, and other developing nations. Cardiovascular research is the key to the prevention, diagnosis, and management of cardiovascular disease. Vigorous and cross-disciplinary approaches are required for successful cardiovascular research. As the boundaries between different scientific disciplines, particularly in the life sciences, are weakening and disappearing, a successful investigator needs to be competent in many different areas, including genetics, cell biology, biochemistry, physiology, and structural biology. The newly developed field of molecular medicine is a cross-disciplinary science that seeks to comprehend disease causes and mechanisms at the molecular level, and to apply this basic research to the prevention, diagnosis, and treatment of diseases and disorders. This volume in the *Methods in Molecular Medicine* series, *Cardiovascular Disease,* provides comprehensive coverage of both basic and the most advanced approaches to the study and characterization of cardiovascular disease. These methods will advance knowledge of the mechanisms, diagnoses, and treatments of cardiovascular disease.

Cardiovascular Disease is a timely volume in which the theory and principles of each method are described in the Introduction section, followed by a detailed description of the materials and equipment needed, and step-by-step protocols for successful execution of the method. A notes section provides advice for potential problems, any modifications, and alternative methods.

We have gathered a group of highly experienced cardiovascular researchers to describe in detail the most important techniques in molecular medicine that are employed in genetic, molecular, cellular, structural, and physiological studies of cardiovascular disease. The thirty-seven chapters in both volumes cover varied methods that include the following:

- Cytogenetic analyses (karyotyping, FISH, array CGH, somatic hybrid analysis).
- Linkage programs for mapping chromosomal locations of disease genes.
- Bioinformatics.
- Human genetics for identifying genes for both monogenic and common complex diseases (positional cloning and genome-wide association study).
- Mouse genetics for identifying genes for complex disease traits (chromosome substitution strains).
- Mutation screening, genetic testing, and high throughput genotyping of single-nucleotide polymorphisms (SNPs).
- Microarray (Genechips) analysis.

- Proteomics.
- Generation of knockout, knock-in, and conditional mutant mice and transgenic overexpression mice for cardiovascular genes.
- Animal models for coronary artery disease, heart failure, hypertension, cardiac arrhythmias, and thrombosis.
- Cardiac physiology (recording techniques for action potentials, sodium and other ionic currents, and optical mapping).
- Cell biology (isolation of adult cardiomyocytes, endothelial cells, smooth muscle cells, angiogenesis, cell proliferation, adhesion, migration, and apoptosis assays).
- Gene transfer and gene therapy (adenovirus vectors, HIV-based retroviral vectors, nucleofection).
- Structural biology (X-ray crystallography, NMR spectroscopy, and electron cryomicroscopy).
- Stem cells.

Cardiovascular Disease should be particularly useful for inspiring undergraduate students, graduate students, postdoctoral fellows, cardiology fellows, clinicians, basic scientists, and other researchers who are entering a new area of cardiovascular research to experience the new challenges. It will serve as a valuable resource book for active researchers when they design new experiments. Although many techniques are described for studying cardiovascular disease, they should be equally valuable for researchers studying other human diseases.

I especially thank Susan De Stefano for her valuable assistance in preparing, reformatting and compiling all the chapters. I also thank Professor John M. Walker, the Series Editor for his invitation to develop this book and his help in editing this book. Finally, I thank all of the authors for the time-consuming job of preparing their chapters.

Qing K. Wang, PhD, MBA

Contents

CONTENTS OF THE COMPANION VOLUME
Volume 2: Molecular Medicine

Contributors

MICHAEL J. ACKERMAN • *Departments of Internal Medicine, Pediatrics and Molecular Pharmacology, and Experimental Therapeutics; Divisions of Cardiovascular Diseases and Pediatric Cardiology, Mayo Clinic College of Medicine, Rochester, MN*

MARK D. ADAMS • *Department of Genetics, Case Western Reserve University, Cleveland, OH*

BLAKE C. BALLIF • *Signature Genomic Laboratories, LLC, Spokane, WA*

BASSEM A. BEJJANI • *Health Research and Education Center, Washington State University, and Signature Genomic Laboratories, LLC, Spokane, WA*

ULRICH BROECKEL • *Department of Medicine, Human and Molecular Genetics Center, Medical College of Wisconsin, Milwaukee, WI*

JEFFREY GULCHER • *Decode Genetics, Reykjavik, Iceland*

BAOCHUAN GUO • *Department of Chemistry, Cleveland State University, Cleveland, OH*

ANNIE E. HILL • *Whitehead Institute for Biomedical Research, Cambridge, MA*

MALGORZATA JARMUZ • *Health Research and Education Center, Washington State University, Spokane, WA*

CATHERINE D. KASHORK • *Signature Genomic Laboratories, LLC, Spokane, WA*

ERIC S. LANDER • *The Broad Institute of MIT and Harvard, Cambridge, MA*

DUANXIANG LI • *Department of Medicine/Cardiology, Oregon Health Science University, Portland, OR*

LIN LI • *Department of Molecular Cardiology, The Cleveland Clinic Foundation, Cleveland, OH*

GEORGE E. LIU • *Bovine Functional Genomics Laboratory, Animal and Natural Resources Institute, US Department of Agriculture-Agriculture Research Service, Beltsville, MD*

ALBERT LUO • *Center for Molecular Genetics, The Cleveland Clinic Foundation, Cleveland, OH*

KAREN MARESSO • *Human and Molecular Genetics Center, Medical College of Wisconsin, Milwaukee, WI*

LISA J. MARTIN • *Department of Pediatrics, Cincinnati Children's Hospital Medical Center and the University of Cincinnati School of Medicine, Cincinnati, OH*

JOSEPH H. NADEAU • *Department of Genetics, Case Western Reserve University School of Medicine, Cleveland, OH*

KOUICHI OZAKI • *RIKEN, SNP Research Center, Tokyo, Japan*

SHAOQI RAO • *Department of Molecular Cardiology, The Cleveland Clinic Foundation, Cleveland, OH*

LISA G. SHAFFER • *Health Research and Education Center, Washington State University and Signature Genomic Laboratories, LLC, Spokane, WA*

GONG-QING SHEN • *Center for Molecular Genetics, The Cleveland Clinic Foundation, Cleveland, OH*

KARI STEFANSSON • *Decode Genetics, Reykjavik, Iceland*

XIYUAN SUN • *Department of Chemistry, Cleveland State University, Cleveland, OH*

TOSHIHIRO TANAKA • *RIKEN, SNP Research Center, Tokyo, Japan*

DAVID J. TESTER • *Departments of Internal Medicine, Pediatrics and Molecular Pharmacology and Experimental Therapeutics; Divisions of Cardiovascular Diseases and Pediatric Cardiology, Mayo Clinic College of Medicine, Rochester, MN*

AARON P. THEISEN • *Health Research and Education Center, Washington State University, Spokane, WA*

AYSE ANIL TIMUR • *Department of Molecular Cardiology, The Cleveland Clinic Foundation, Cleveland, OH*

QING K. WANG • *Department of Molecular Cardiology, Center for Cardiovascular Genetics, Department of Cardiovascular Medicine, The Cleveland Clinic Foundation, Cleveland, OH*

MELISSA L. WILL • *Departments of Internal Medicine, Pediatrics and Molecular Pharmacology & Experimental Therapeutics; Divisions of Cardiovascular Diseases and Pediatric Cardiology, Mayo Clinic College of Medicine, Rochester, MN*

1

Cytogenetic Analysis of Cardiovascular Disease

Karyotyping

Malgorzata Jarmuz and Lisa G. Shaffer

Summary

Numerical and structural chromosomal rearrangements, such as aneuploidies, deletions, duplications, and other aberrations have been associated with congenital abnormalities, pregnancy loss, and malignancy. Detection of these genetic changes is possible by cytogenetic analysis. The karyotype is determined by analysis of metaphase or prometaphase chromosomes of peripheral blood lymphocytes after banding procedures. This analysis plays an important role in determining patient diagnosis and care. In this chapter, we describe the basic approach of cytogenetic analysis: arresting the cell in metaphase or prometaphase, the obtaining of metaphase chromosome spreads, and staining and chromosome analysis.

Key Words: GTG banding; karyotype; chromosomal aberration.

1. Introduction

Karyotype analysis after chromosome banding is the standard method for identifying numerical and structural chromosome aberrations in cytogenetic diagnosis. The technique was introduced in the 1970s and has become an integral part of the diagnostic workup for chromosome alterations in congenital disorders and cancer conditions. The efficiency and broad application of classical cytogenetics made it an important tool in research diagnostics. Although the main limitation of classical cytogenetics is its inability to detect structural rearrangements smaller than 5 Mb in routine analysis *(1)*, this problem has been overcome with the establishment of newer techniques of molecular cytogenetics (e.g., fluorescence *in situ* hybridization [FISH]). The combination of cytogenetics with molecular methods resolves many of the problems encountered in clinical diagnosis. Collectively, cytogenetics remains a powerful tech-

From: *Methods in Molecular Medicine, Vol. 128: Cardiovascular Disease; Methods and Protocols; Volume 1*
Edited by: Q. Wang © Humana Press Inc., Totowa, NJ

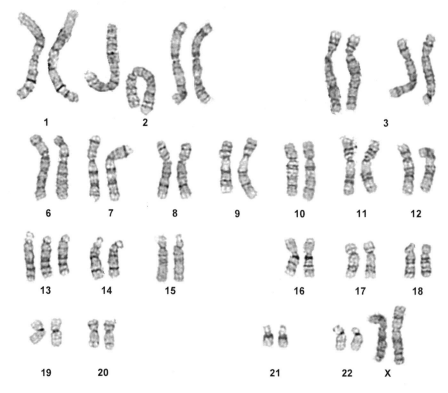

Fig. 1. Karyotype showing trisomy 13, indicated by the extra copy of chromosome 13.

nique in medical and research laboratories for identifying and understanding chromosome abnormalities.

Chromosomal abnormalities are among the genetic causes of cardiovascular disease. Congenital heart defects occur in many chromosomal syndromes, including Down syndrome (trisomy 21 or partial duplication of the long arm of chromosome 21), trisomy 13 (**Fig. 1**) and 18, monosomy X, DiGeorge/velocardiofacial syndrome (microscopic or submicroscopic deletion of chromosome band 22q11.2), Williams syndrome (submicroscopic deletion of band 7q11.23), and many other unbalanced chromosomal rearrangements *(2–5)*.

Chromosomes may be obtained from many different kinds of tissues, but peripheral blood is the most easily acquired human tissue. Because blood lymphocytes can produce a large quantity of good-quality mitoses, they are an ideal substrate for the determination of constitutional karyotypes. They are also amenable to synchronization, which is important for high-resolution analysis of chromosomes. A basic assumption is that karyotypes of blood cells are representative of other somatic cells of an individual. However, mosaicism, the presence of two or more chromosomally distinct cell lines, should also be considered. For this reason, analysis of other tissues may be required to exclude or identify mosaicism.

Chromosome analysis is performed on dividing cells. To stimulate cell division, lymphocytes from peripheral blood require a mitotic agent such as phytohemagglutinin (PHA) or pokeweed antigen *(6,7)*. PHA primarily stimulates the T-cell population of lymphocytes to enter the cell cycle and go through mitosis, whereas pokeweed stimulates the B-cell population. PHA is the most commonly used mitogen for stimulated cultures of peripheral blood. During the first 24 h of exposure to this antigen, T lymphocytes dedifferentiate to T-lymphoblastic cells, which have the ability to synthesize DNA and undergo mitosis. The optimum harvesting point for cytogenetic analysis is after 60–70 h of culture, but it may range from 48 h (particularly for newborns) to 96 h, when an adequate number of mitotic cells can be produced for analysis *(8)*.

To obtain longer, high-resolution prophase or prometaphase chromosomes, the synchronization of the cell cycle in culture, combined with anti-chromosomal contraction additives, must be applied. Synchronization is accomplished by blocking mitoses during DNA synthesis using chemicals such as methotrexate, thymidine (TdR), fluorodeoxyuridine (FudR), or bromodeoxyuridine (BrdU) during the last 16–18 h of culture. The block is released with thymidine (for methotrexate or BrdU), bromodeoxyuridine (for methotrexate), 2-deoxycytidine (for thymidine), or washing cells in medium and further reculture of cells in medium without PHA. The release time varies from 4.5 h to approx 5 h. This is the time required for completion of the S, G_2, and mitotic phases of the cell cycle. During this time, 1–2 h before harvesting, a chemical preventing normal chromosome contraction by binding to or intercalating into DNA or chromatin (e.g., ethidium bromide, actinomycin D, Hoest 33258) should be added *(7)*.

Mitotic chromosomes are obtained by treating cultures with colcemid, a mitotic arrestant that inhibits spindle fiber formation in the dividing cells *(9)* and, thus, prohibits the sister chromatids from moving to opposite poles to form two daughter cells. Mitotic arrest is followed by treatment with a hypotonic solution to increase cell volume. The final steps are the fixation of cells with methanol/acetic acid to remove water and to kill and preserve the chromosomes prior to the banding procedures. G-banding using trypsin and Giemsa stain (GTG banding) is the most frequently used banding technique in clinical laboratories. This banding technique produces a series of light and dark transverse bands along the lengths of chromosomes, which permit the identification of chromosomes and their regions.

2. Materials

2.1. Specimen

Whole blood (about 5 mL for adults and 2 mL for infants) should be collected in a sodium heparin (*see* **Note 1**) sterile tube. Because live cells are required for culturing of cells, the specimen should be provided to a laboratory within 24 h. Room temperature (no less than 4°C) is recommended for shipping and storage.

2.2. Tissue Culture

1. Complete medium RPMI 1640 (can be stored for 4 wk in 4°C): 87 mL of RPMI 1640, 10 mL of fetal bovine serum (FBS), 1 mL L-glutamine, 1 mL penicillin/ streptomycin (or other antibiotic for example gentamycin).
2. Complete medium RPMI must be supplemented with PHA, 1 mg/mL, for blood culture. Fresh PHA should be prepared every 2 wk by adding 5 mL deionized water to 5 mg lyophilized PHA (stored at 4°C). The medium and PHA should be pretested for sterility and amenability to growth.

2.3. Harvesting

1. Fluorodeoxyuridine (FudR; 5-Fluoro-2'-Deoxyuridine): dissolve 0.0246 g FudR in 10 mL deionized water to make a 10^{-2} M FudR solution. Add 1 mL of 10^{-2} M FudR to 9 mL deionized water to prepare 10^{-4} M or 2.46 µg/mL of working solution. Sterilize by filtration under the laminar flow hood. Protect from light. Store at –15 to –20°C. The solution can be stored up to 1 yr.
2. Thymidine (TdR): dissolve 0.25 g TdR in 10 mL deionized water to make a 0.1 M working solution. Sterilize by filtration under the laminar flow hood. Protect from light. Store at –15 to –20°C. The solution can be stored up to 1 yr.
3. Ethidium bromide (EB): prepare 1 mg/mL working solution. Sterilize by filtration under the laminar flow hood. Protect from light. Store at 4°C. (EB is carcinogenic and should be handled with care.)
4. Colcemid® solution, 10 µg/mL. Colcemid is a toxic chemical. Avoid skin contact.
5. Hypotonic solution: 0.075 M potassium chloride (KCl) (warm to 37°C before use).
6. Fixative: mix one part of glacial acetic acid to three parts absolute methanol (freshly prepared). Fixative is toxic, corrosive and flammable. Avoid skin contact.

2.4. GTG Banding

1. Giemsa stain. Store at room temperature.
2. Citrate-phosphate buffer, pH 6.8: 22.35 g of Na_2HPO_4 and 4.47 g of citric acid, dissolve in 1000 mL deionized H_2O. Store at 4°C.
3. Enzar-T trypsin, 40X concentrate. Store at –20°C.
4. 7.5% sodium bicarbonate ($NaHCO_3$). Store at 4°C.
5. Hank's balanced salt solution (HBSS), 1X solution, without Ca^{++} and Mg^{++}, with phenol red, pH 7.0–7.2. Store at room temperature.
6. Distilled water.

3. Methods

3.1. Tissue Culture

Peripheral blood can be cultured in different commercially available media. A medium for optimal cell division must contain amino acids, carbohydrates, vitamins, buffered salts, and an antibiotic to prevent bacterial contaminations and should have a constant pH. For blood cultures, a mitogen used to stimulate division of T lymphocytes is added to complete medium.

The correct temperature, pH, and CO_2 level are important for blood culture. The optimal temperature for culturing of blood is 37°C. The ideal pH level is between 7.2 and 7.4; pH is maintained in an open culture system in an incubator with a controlled CO_2 level of 5%. Otherwise, a closed cultured system should be used. Work in a laminar flow hood (*see* **Note 2**).

1. Prepare RPMI medium with PHA: to prepare 10 mL medium add 0.1 mL PHA to 9.9 mL complete RPMI.
2. Prepare four 15-mL conical tubes or T25 flasks with media, two for cultures with no additives and one each for the addition of TdR and FudR. Add 5 mL complete medium to each tube and 0.4 mL whole blood for adults and 0.3 mL for infants to each tube.
3. Recap culture tubes, mix blood with media, and place in an incubator at 37°C for 48–96 h. The optimal incubation time is 72 h for adults and 48 h for children less than 3 mo old. The tubes should be kept at a 45° angle to provide an increased surface area. If the culture is in 25-cm flasks with open caps, the incubator must have atmospheric CO_2 at 5%.

3.2. Harvesting

Three basic steps comprise the harvesting procedure: the addition of colcemid (mitotic arrestant), incubation in hypotonic solution, and fixation. If the culture tubes are being prepared only for routine harvesting, start from **step 7**.

1. One Day before harvest, add 50 µL working solution of TdR to one culture and 50 µL working solution of FudR to a different culture.
2. Day of harvest: 17–17.5 h after adding the TdR and FudR to two separate cultures, invert these tubes to mix well and centrifuge at 440*g* for 5 min. If grown in flasks, cultures must be transferred to 15-mL conical tubes before centrifugation.
3. Remove and discard the supernatant, lightly tap pellet, and add 5 mL of RPMI medium (unsupplemented). Recap tubes and invert to mix well and centrifuge at 440*g* for 5 min.
4. Discard supernatant and add 5 mL of RPMI medium. Recap the tubes, mix well by inversion and reincubate for 3 h and 10 min.
5. Add 30 µL of EB to cultures previously grown in the presence of TdR and FudR and incubate at 37°C for 1 h and 45 min.
6. Prewarm the hypotonic solution at 37°C.
7. Add 50 µL of Colcemid (*see* **Note 3**) to the cultures. Incubate for 10–20 min in

the 37°C incubator. The optimal incubation time to achieve the desired chromosome length must be determined in each laboratory.

8. Remove tubes from incubator and centrifuge at 440*g* for 10 min.
9. Discard supernatant (do not disturb the top layer of the pellet; *see* **Note 4**), lightly tap cell pellets to loosen them, and add 2 mL hypotonic solution to each tube. After each pellet has been exposed to hypotonic, add an additional 10 mL hypotonic to each tube, mix well but gently (*see* **Note 5**) by Pasteur pipet, recap, and gently invert tubes several times.
10. Incubate 20 min at room temperature.
11. Prepare fresh fixative (*see* **Note 6**). At the end of the 20-min incubation, slowly add about 2 mL of fixative to each tube and mix.
12. Centrifuge at 800*g* for 7 min.
13. Discard supernatant, lightly tap pellet to resuspend the cells, add 5 mL fixative to each tube (the first 1–2 mL dropwise), and mix well.
14. Incubate 15 min in room temperature.
15. Centrifuge at 800*g* for 7 min.
16. Remove supernatant and tap tube gently to mix pellet, add 5 mL fixative, and mix well. Centrifuge for 7 min at 800*g*.
17. Repeat **step 10**. Store pellets in the freezer if slides are not being prepared immediately (*see* **Note 7**).

3.3. Chromosome Slide Preparation

Slide making is the least understood and standardized step of karyotyping. Several variables affect the preparation of good-quality slides. The preparation of slides can be highly dependent on humidity and temperature and the experience and skill of the individual making the slides.

Slides for chromosome analysis are prepared from cell pellets harvested from lymphocyte cultures:

1. Clean microscope slides: store microscope slides in absolute ethanol or purified water. If stored in ethanol, rinse slides in purified water before using.
2. Prepare fresh fixative.
3. Centrifuge the harvest pellet at 800*g* for 5 min, discard supernatant, and resuspend the pellet in fresh fix to make a slightly cloudy suspension.
4. Apply five to eight drops of fresh fix to the slide and allow to drain off, then apply one to three drops of cell suspension while holding the slide at a 30–45° angle to allow the suspension to run off the slide. Place the slide at a 30° angle against the tube rack and allow it to dry (*see* **Note 8**).
5. Observe the slide using a phase contrast microscope to assess the suspension density, the spreading of the chromosomes, and chromosome morphology.
   a. Cell density: the proper concentration of the cell fixative suspension is very important to slide preparation. If the suspension is too diluted, it will be difficult to find mitotic cells. In this event, centrifuge and resuspend in less fixative. If the suspension is too dense, it will inhibit chromosome spreading. In

this event, dilute the cell suspension with fixative.

b. Degree of spreading: the goal is obtain uniform dispersal of chromosomes. Chromosomes should be well spaced, but not overspread (broken metaphases cannot be analyzed with confidence) and with a minimal number of overlapping chromosomes.

c. Chromosome morphology: the chromosomes should appear flat, with sharp chromosome margins and a minimum of cytoplasm for subsequent good quality bands.

3.4. G-Banding Using Trypsin and Giemsa Stain

1. Prepare aged slides: place prepared slides in an oven at 90°C for 35 min if slides were prepared the same day or at 90°C for 25 min if the slides have aged at room temperature overnight or longer (*see* **Note 9**).
2. Prepare five coplin jars with the following solutions:

   a. 50 mL HBSS (1X).

   b. 50 mL HBSS + 0.2 mL Enzar-T trypsin (adjust pH to 7.0–7.2 with $NaHCO_3$).

   c. 70% ethanol.

   d. 70% ethanol.

   e. 50 mL deionized water + 2 mL citrate-phosphate buffer + 2 mL Giemsa stain.

3. In a separate jar, place about 300 mL H_2O for rinsing slides after staining.
4. Place up to four slides in HBSS (jar 1) for 3–5 min.
5. Transfer one slide (never band all the slides on one patient in a single run) to trypsin (jar 2) to determine optimal trypsinization time (*see* **Note 10**). The trypsinization time should be the same for slides prepared at the same time and in the same way from the same patient. Prepare three to five identical slides for analysis.
6. Transfer slide to the first ethanol solution (jar 3), followed by the second ethanol solution (jar 4). Remo ˝ slide and let drain briefly, removing excess ethanol from the back of the slide.
7. Place slide in Giemsa stain (jar 5) for 5–8 min.
8. Rinse slide in water.
9. Dry slide using air from a compressed air source.
10. Examine the slide under a microscope, using a dry (non-oil) objective, to assess banding. Adjust banding if necessary. Select cells which are well spread and have good length; these cells will be examined during analysis. If the chromosomes are pale and difficult to see under low power, they have been understained; increase the stain time by 2–3 min. If the chromosomes are dark and solid-stained, they have been overstained; the trypsin time may need to be increased. However, because it is difficult to overstain in 5–8 min, if the slides are dark and solid-stained it is likely that an error has been made in the preparation of the solutions. Prepare new solutions and repeat the procedure with the next slide. If the bands are not visible on the chromosomes, increase the trypsinization time. If the chromosomes are fuzzy in appearance or look "chewed," reduce the trypsinization time.
11. When the correct trypsinization time and stain time have been established, two to four slides can be banded at the same time.

3.5. Chromosome Analysis

At least 20 banded metaphases should be counted and examined. In case of suspected mosaicism or a study to exclude mosaicism, the count should be increased to 30 or higher depending on the extent of mosaicism one is trying to exclude. Band level is important during analysis: for detection of trisomies, 400 bands per haploid set (BPHS) is adequate to exclude aneuploidy, but 550–850 BPHS is necessary to detect most structural rearrangements. At least five metaphase cells should be examined in detail (comparing the homologues band for band). The final results should be described using the nomenclature outlined in International System for Human Cytogenetic Nomenclature 2005 *(10)*. Guidelines for the clinical analysis of banded chromosomes can be obtained from the American College of Medical Genetics (http://www.acmg.net/Pages/ACMG_Activities/stds-2002/e.htm).

4. Notes

1. Other anticoagulants such as lithium heparin and EDTA can be toxic to dividing cells.
2. Although bacterial contamination of blood culture is rare, an aseptic technique should be employed at all stages of culture initiation.
3. Colcemid timing is very important: excessive time with colcemid will produce high mitotic index but short chromosomes, whereas insufficient time will result in a low mitotic index that may not be sufficient for analysis.
4. Disrupting the top layer of the pellet can be the cause of a low mitotic index and/or small pellet. A small amount of excess supernatant cell pellet is recommended.
5. Gentle but thorough mixing of the pellets is important at each step.
6. Fixative should not be prepared before hypotonic stage and fixative should not be added before hypotonic solution; in the latter situation, the result will be a total loss of a harvest.
7. Cells should be stored as pellets rather than suspended in fixative.
8. Making slides is the most critical step in chromosome preparation for chromosome analysis. If the slides are well prepared, the subsequent steps of G-banding and chromosome analysis can be performed more easily.
9. Check the temperature before aging slides. Changes in aging conditions will affect the banding quality.
10. Do not agitate the jars while slides are in trypsin or stain.

References

1. Shaffer, L. G., Ledbetter, D. H., and Lupski, J. R. (2001) Molecular cytogenetics of contiguous gene syndromes: mechanism and consequences of gene dosage imbalance, in *Metabolic and Molecular Basis of Inherited Disease,* (Scriver, C. R., Beaudet, A., Sly, W. S., et al., eds.), McGraw Hill, NJ, pp.1291–1324.

2. Gelb, B. D. (2001) Genetic basis of syndromes associated with congenital heart disease. *Curr. Opin. Cardiol.* **16,** 188–194.

3. Gelb, B. D. (2000) Recent advances in the understanding of genetic causes of congenital heart defects. *Front Biosci.* **1,** D321–D333.

4. van Karnebeek, C. D. and Hennekam, R. C. (1999) Associations between chromosomal anomalies and congenital heart defects: a database search. *Am. J. Med. Genet.* **84,** 158–166.

5. Tennstedt, C., Chaoui, R., Korner, H., and Dietel, M. (1999) Spectrum of congenital heart defects and extracardiac malformations associated with chromosomal abnormalities: results of a seven year necropsy study. *Heart* **82,** 34–39.

6. Nowell, P. C. (1960) Phytohemagglutinin: an initiator of mitosis in cultures of normal human leukocytes. *Cancer Res.* **20,** 462–466.

7. Barch, M. J., Knutsen, T., and Spurbeck, J. L. (1997) *The AGT Cytogenetics Laboratory Manual,* Lippincott-Raven, Philadelphia, NJ.

8. Michalowski, A. (1963) Time-course of DNA synthesis in human leukocyte cultures. *Exp. Cell Res.* **32,** 609–612.

9. Taylor, E. W. (1965) The mechanism of colchicine inhibition of mitosis. I. Kinetics of inhibition and the binding of h3-colchicine. *Cell Biol.* **25(Suppl),** 145–160.

10. Shaffer, C. G. and Tommerup, N. (2005) *ISCN (2005): An International System for Human Cytogenetic Nomenclature,* S. Karger, Basel, Switzerland.

2

Fluorescence *In Situ* Hybridization in Cardiovascular Disease

Ayse Anil Timur and Qing K. Wang

Summary

Many human diseases are associated with cytogenetic abnormalities or chromosomal disorders including translocations, deletions, duplications, inversions, and other complicated chromosomal changes. Fluorescence *in situ* hybridization (FISH), a technique involving hybridization of labeled probes to chromosomes and detection of hybridization via fluorochromes, has become a popular method for identification and characterization of cytogenetic abnormalities. For FISH analysis, metaphase chromosomes are prepared by mitotic arrest and hypotonic shock, and denatured. Hybridization of digoxigenin- or biotin-labeled probes to these chromosomes is visualized using fluorochromes like fluorescein isothiocyanate and Texas Red. We have successfully applied FISH technology to the characterization of chromosome breakpoints involved in disease-associated cytogenetic abnormalities to identify candidate gene(s) for the disease. FISH is also widely used in clinical diagnosis of chromosomal disorders.

Key Words: Fluorescence *in situ* hybridization; FISH; chromosome painting probes; metaphase chromosomes; cytogenetic abnormality; chromosomal disorder; disease.

1. Introduction

In situ hybridization is a technique for visualizing target nucleic acid sequences on chromosomes by using complementary probe sequences. The technique is called fluorescence *in situ* hybridization (FISH) when fluorescent detection is utilized. This technology has been applied to many clinical and research studies such as identification of chromosomal abnormalities, comparative cytogenetics, gene mapping, characterization of somatic cell hybrids, and positional cloning. FISH involves the cellular preparation of chromosomes, labeling of probes, hybridization of labeled probes to chromosomes, and detection of the hybridization signals. The chromosomal targets for FISH vary from

From: *Methods in Molecular Medicine, Vol. 128: Cardiovascular Disease; Methods and Protocols; Volume 1*
Edited by: Q. Wang © Humana Press Inc., Totowa, NJ

metaphase chromosomes to extended strands of DNA *(1)*. Hybridized probes can be localized on a highly defined genetic map. High-resolution metaphase chromosomes can be used to resolve two sequences approx 1 Mb apart, whereas interphase mapping allows the resolution of sequences 100 kb apart. Using extended DNA fibers, sequences 1 kb apart can also be resolved *(2)*.

Metaphase chromosomes can be prepared from any population of actively dividing cells by treating cells first with colcemid or vinblastine to arrest mitosis and then with a hypotonic KCl solution to increase cellular volume. The cells are then fixed with methanol/acetic acid to remove water and disrupt cell membranes before being spread onto microscope slides.

A variety of probes targeting repetitive or unique sequences on the chromosomes can be used for FISH. Centromeres and telomeres of mammalian chromosomes usually contain large arrays of simple DNA motifs that produce strong signals with FISH. Unique probes can be prepared from PCR products, cDNAs, cloned genomic DNAs such as cosmids, P1 artificial chromosomes (PACs), bacterial artificial chromosomes (BACs), and yeast artificial chromosomes (YACs). Labeling of YAC DNA is often problematic, and a large amount of probe is required. *Alu*-PCR amplification of total yeast DNA increases the yield of YAC DNA probe and, therefore, hybridization efficiency *(3)*. Whole-chromosome or chromosome-arm painting probes are also available for human chromosomes. These are derived from flow-sorted chromosomes, either as pooled clones from chromosome-specific libraries or by PCR amplification *(4)*. Repetitive sequences in large DNA probes and chromosome paints will result in unspecific hybridization signals all over the genome and should be suppressed with an unlabeled human competitor DNA, such as sonicated total human DNA or *Cot-1* DNA *(5)*.

FISH probes can be labeled directly or indirectly by fluorochromes. They are generally labeled indirectly with digoxigenin (DIG)- or biotin-conjugated to dUTP. Nick translation is the most widely used method for the labeling of probes *(6)*. After hybridization of labeled probes to chromosomes, fluorescent detection of hybridization is carried out using anti-DIG or anti-biotin antibodies conjugated to fluorochromes. The most frequently used dyes are fluorescein isothiocyanate (FITC), which emits a green fluorescence, or dyes with red or orange fluorescence, Texas Red and Cy3 *(7)*. For probes labeled directly using dUTP conjugated with a fluorochrome, there is no need for a further detection procedure. For FISH experiments, chromosomes and cell nuclei are also counterstained by a fluorescent dye that is specific for DNA. The most commonly used dye is 4',6-diamidino-2-phenyl-indol (DAPI), which is excited in the ultraviolet and with which chromosomes and cell nuclei show a bright blue fluorescence. DAPI also gives a G-banded pattern to chromosomes.

Analysis of the FISH results is carried out under a fluorescence microscope connected with a cooled charge-coupled device (CCD) camera.

In our laboratory, we use metaphase chromosomes for the characterization of chromosomes of the somatic hybrids and localization of chromosomal breakpoints to identify candidate gene(s) for several human disorders *(8,9)*. Metaphase chromosome spreads are prepared from mouse–human hybrid cells and/or human lymphoblastoid cells. YAC and BAC DNAs containing our target sequences are used to prepare probes for FISH. Probes are generally labeled with DIG and hybridization signals are detected using an anti-DIG antibody conjugated with FITC.

2. Materials

2.1. Preparation of Metaphase Chromosomes

1. Suspension or attached cell cultures (*see* **Note 1**).
2. Dulbecco's modified Eagle's medium (DMEM) supplemented with 10% fetal bovine serum (FBS) and 1X antibiotic-antimycotic solution (Gibco BRL), prewarmed to 37°C (*see* **Note 2**).
3. Phosphate-buffered saline (PBS) solution, prewarmed to 37°C (*see* **Note 3**).
4. Trypsin/EDTA solution: 5% (w/v) trypsin, 2% (w/v) EDTA, prewarmed to 37°C.
5. Vinblastine (Sigma) (*see* **Note 4**).
6. Hypotonic solution: 0.075 M KCl, prewarmed to 37°C (*see* **Note 5**).
7. Fixative: 3:1 (v/v) methanol/glacial acetic acid, ice-cold (*see* **Note 6**).
8. 15-mL conical-bottom plastic tubes.

2.2. Preparation of Chromosome Slides

1. Fixative: 3:1 (v/v) methanol/glacial acetic acid, ice-cold.
2. Microscope slides (one end frosted) (*see* **Note 7**).
3. Micropipet.
4. Lint-free tissue (Kimwipes).
5. Standard phase-contrast microscope.

2.3. Preparation of Probes

1. 500 ng of probe DNAs (*see* **Note 8**).
2. DIG- and/or biotin-nick translation mix (Roche) (*see* **Note 9**).
3. Human *Cot-1* DNA (Invitrogen) and sonicated human placental DNA (Sigma) (*see* **Note 10**).
4. 5 M NaCl.
5. Ice-cold absolute ethanol.
6. 70% ethanol.
7. Hybridization buffer: 50% (v/v) deionized formamide, 10% (w/v) dextran sulfate, 1% (v/v) Tween-20, 2X SSC, pH 7.0 (*see* **Note 11**).

8. Chromosome painting probes (optional) (*see* **Note 12**).
9. Heat block or PCR machine.

2.4. In Situ *Hybridization*

1. 2X SSC, pH 7.0, prewarmed to 37°C.
2. 70, 85, and 100% ethanol.
3. Coplin jars.
4. Water bath.
5. HYBrite (Vysis) denaturation/hybridization unit (*see* **Note 13**).
6. Cover slips.

2.5. Detection of Hybridization

1. Solution I: 50% (v/v) formamide, 2X SSC, pH 7.0, prewarmed to 43°C (*see* **Note 14**).
2. Solution II: 0.6X SSC, pH 7.0, prewarmed to 50°C.
3. Solution III: 4X SSC, 0.1% (v/v) Tween-20, pH 7.0.
4. Solution IV: 5% (w/v) nonfat dry milk (*see* **Note 15**).
5. Solution V: 2X SSC, pH 7.0, room temperature.
6. Anti-DIG or Anti-biotin antibodies conjugated with fluorochromes (*see* **Note 16**).
7. Mounting medium with DAPI (VECTASHIELD, Vector laboratories).
8. Light protective Eppendorf tubes.
9. Parafilm.

3. Methods

3.1. Preparation of Metaphase Chromosomes From Suspension and Attached Cells

1. Cells are split at 60–80% confluence 1 d before the preparation of metaphase chromosomes. The next day, 10 mL of fresh medium is added to the suspension cells. For attached cells, 5 mL of old medium in a tissue-culture plate is replaced with 10 mL of fresh medium. Cells are incubated for 5–6 h in a humidified 37°C, 10% CO_2 incubator (*see* **Note 17**).
2. Vinblastine is directly added to the cell media to a final concentration of 1 μg/mL and cells are returned to the incubator for a further 30 min (*see* **Note 18**).
3. Suspension cells are directly transferred into a 15-mL conical-bottom plastic tube. For attached cells, a modest trypsinization combined with a sharp tap on the culture plate is carried out to collect the rounded, mitotic cells.
4. Cells are centrifuged for 5 min at 400g. Supernatant (medium) is removed completely except for about 300 μL. Cell pellet is resuspended in this volume by flicking.
5. 10 mL of 0.075 *M* KCl is added and cells are incubated in a 37°C water bath for 4 min for the human lymphoblastoid cells and for 15 min for the mouse–human hybrids (*see* **Note 19**).
6. Cells are centrifuged for 5 min at 400g.

7. Supernatant is removed except for about 300 μL. Cell pellet is resuspended in this volume by flicking.
8. A few drops of ice-cold fixative (methanol:acetic acid, 3:1) is added to the cells and flicked gently several times. Then, another 8 mL of the fixative solution is added.
9. Cells are centrifuged for 5 min at 400g.
10. Supernatant is aspirated and cell pellet is resuspended in 5–8 mL of the methanol-acetic acid solution. Cells should be restored at –20°C at least for 1–2 h before use (*see* **Note 20**).

3.2. Preparation of Chromosome Spreads

1. Microscope slides kept in a container filled with 70% ethanol are dried up.
2. By tilting the slide to 30–45°, 5–10 μL of cell suspension is dropped from a height of about 5–7 in. onto the part close to the frosted end of the slide, then the slide is immediately tilted more to allow the cell solution spread down through the slide surface. Slides are left to air-dry and chromosome spreads are examined under a microscope (*see* **Notes 21** and **22**).

3.3. Labeling and Denaturation of Probes

1. Probe labeling is carried out on ice in a 10-μL reaction volume. Water is used to complete the volume. 500 ng of probe DNA is mixed with 2 μL of DIG- or biotin-nick translation mix (Roche, Applied Science) on ice.
2. Reaction mixture is incubated at 15°C for 90 min.
3. Reaction is stopped by heating the mixture to 65°C for 10 min.
4. Whole reaction volume (10 μL) is mixed with 5 μg of *Cot-1* DNA, 1 μg of human placental DNA, and 0.02 vol 5 M NaCl in a volume of 50 μL completed with water. 125 μL of ice-cold ethanol (2.5 vol) is added and mixture is kept at –20°C for 30 min.
5. Mixture is centrifuged for 25 min at the maximum speed in a microcentrifuge.
6. 100 μL of 70% ethanol is added to the pellet and centrifuged for 10 min at the maximum speed.
7. Supernatant is removed very carefully and 15 μL of hybridization buffer:water (7:3) is immediately added without letting the pellet to dry up. Allow DNA to dissolve at room temperature for 30 min to 1 h (*see* **Note 23**).
8. Chromosome painting probes can be added to the precipitated, labeled probe at this stage (*see* **Note 24**).
9. The labeled probe is denatured at 70°C for 10 min and reannealed at 37°C for 30 min, and kept on ice until ready to add chromosome slides.

3.4. Chromosome Denaturation and Hybridization

1. Chromosome slides are placed in coplin jars and 2X SSC, pH 7.0, prewarmed to 37°C is added. They are incubated in 37°C water bath for 30–45 min.
2. Slides are dehydrated through ethanol series of 70, 85, and 100% for 1 min each and air-dried.

3. 15 µL of hybridization buffer:water (7:3) mixture is placed longitudinally onto the slide following the mid-line; put a cover slip on it by avoiding air bubbles between cover slip and slide (*see* **Note 25**).
4. Slides are placed onto the plate of HYBrite; chromosomes are denatured at 70°C for 1 min (*see* **Note 26**). They are immediately put on ice (*see* **Note 27**).
5. The cover slip is removed carefully, the previously labeled probe is placed longitudinally on the slide following the mid-line, and a cover slip is placed on it, with no air bubbles allowed between the cover slip and slide.
6. Slides are placed onto the HYBrite plate and left for incubation at 37°C overnight (*see* **Note 28**).

3.5. Detection of Hybridization Signals

1. Cover slips are removed gently by dipping the slides in solution I once, and then slides are washed three times in solution I for 5 min each in a 43°C water bath (*see* **Note 29**).
2. Slides are washed three times in solution II for 7 min each in a 50°C water bath.
3. Slides are equilibrated in solution III for 3 min at room temperature.
4. Long sheets of Parafilm are cut to cover the bottom of a container. 120 µL of solution IV per slide is placed for each slide on these Parafilm sheets.
5. Slides from the solution III are drained by touching the short edge of the slide to a lint-free tissue and covered onto each 120 µL solution IV, which was placed on the Parafilm. The container is humidified (*see* **Note 28**) and slides are incubated for 10 min at room temperature.
6. While slides are incubating, antibodies conjugated with fluorochromes are diluted with solution IV in sufficient amounts (120 µL of the diluted antibodies per slide) (*see* **Note 30**). Dilution is carried out in a light-protective Eppendorf tube and centrifuge for 5 min at the maximum speed in a microcentrifuge to eliminate some participation particles.
7. Slides are removed from the chamber and placed upside down in a safe place, and the old Parafilm sheets are replaced with the new ones. 120 µL of the antibody-conjugated fluorochrome solution is placed for each slide on these new Parafilm sheets.
8. Slides are covered onto each 120 µL antibody-conjugated fluorochrome solution that was placed on the Parafilm. The container is humidified (*see* **Note 28**) and wrapped with foil. Slides are incubated 30 min at a 37°C incubator.
9. Slides are washed in solution III three times for 5 min each in dark at room temperature.
10. Slides are washed finally in solution V once for 5 min in the dark at room temperature.
11. Slides are lined up on a lint-free tissue at an angle to let them drain. Two drops of DAPI are placed on the middle of each slide, and the slides are covered with cover slips. Excess DAPI is removed by placing the slide between towel sheets and gently pressing on top. They can be kept in slide boxes for several weeks at 4 or –20°C. Now, the slides are ready to be examined under a fluorescence microscope. Because there are two sister chromatids, hybridization signals are gener-

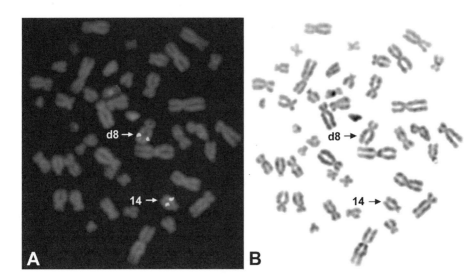

Fig. 1. Localization of translocation t(8;14) (q22.3;q13) breakpoints by fluorescence *in situ* hybridization (FISH) analysis. (**A**) *Alu*-PCR product of yeast artificial chromosome (YAC) 964b11 (from chromosome 14) DNA was labeled by digoxigenin (DIG)-nick translation and hybridized to metaphase chromosome spreads prepared from the lymphoblastoid cells of a patient with Klippel-Trenaunay syndrome (KTS). This patient with KTS carries a balanced translocation involving chromosomes 8 and 14 *(8)*. Hybridization signals were detected using an anti-DIG antibody conjugated with FITC, which gives a green fluorescence as pointed by arrows. Biotin-labeled chromosome 14q arm-specific painting probe was used as a marker and hybridization was detected by using Texas red, which gives a pinkish to red color. Metaphase chromosomes were counterstained by DAPI showing blue fluorescence. Because green hybridization signals were detected only on the normal chromosome 14 and derivative chromosome 8 (d8), the chromosome 14 translocation breakpoint should be located above the position of this YAC clone. (**B**) The same image as in A was processed for G-banding patterns.

ally seen as two dots on the metaphase chromosomes. An example of the FISH data is shown in **Fig. 1**.

4. Notes

1. In our laboratory, metaphase chromosomes are prepared from the suspension cultures of human lymphoblastoid cells and attached cultures of mouse–human hybrid cells. Lymphoblastoid cells are maintained in 25-cm^2 cell-culture flasks and hybrid cells are grown in 100-mm tissue-culture plates.
2. For antibiotic-antimycotic, 100X solution is purchased from Invitrogen. It contains 10,000 U/mL penicillin G sodium, 10,000 μg/mL streptomycin sulfate, and 25 μg/mL amphotericin B.
3. All PBS solutions mentioned here contain 137 m*M* of NaCl, 2.7 m*M* of KCl,

8.0 mM of Na$_2$HPO$_4$-7H$_2$O, and 1.5 mM of KH$_2$PO$_4$.

4. Vinblastine can be purchased from Sigma as 5 mg powder. It is dissolved in 5 mL of PBS to a stock solution of 1 mg/mL and kept at 4°C in dark.

5. KCl can be prepared as 0.75 M stock solution and, prior to the experiment, can be diluted to 0.075 M with sterile water.

6. Fixative solution should be prepared fresh each time and kept at –20°C.

7. Microscope slides are placed on slide racks, and the racks are placed in a big container filled with water and a detergent suitable for glassware. The container is placed on a shaker for 15 min; then, the slides are rinsed with distilled water several times following a final 15-min rinse on the shaker. Finally, racks are kept in a big container filled with 70% ethanol.

8. Our probes for FISH are prepared from YAC and BAC DNAs. YAC probes are prepared by *Alu*-PCR specifically using 200–400 ng of YAC DNA, 0.5 µM of *Alu*-specific ALE1 primer (5'-GCCTCCCAAAGTGCTGGGATTACAG-3') and ALE3 primer (5'-CCA[C/T]TGCACTCCAGCCTGGG-3'), and 4 mM of MgCl$_2$. PCR products are purified using QIAquick spin columns (QIAquick PCR purification kit, Qiagen Inc.).

9. We generally label our probes with DIG and use chromosome painting probes labeled with Biotin.

10. Human *Cot-1* DNA and total human placental DNA is used to suppress cross-hybridization of large human DNA probes to the human repetitive DNA sequences.

11. Dextran sulfate used in the preparation of hybridization buffer is difficult to dissolve. After adding all ingredients, the preparation should be kept in a 70°C water bath for several hours and then allowed to cool down. The pH of the solution is adjusted to 7.0 and its volume is brought to the desired value. It is sterilized by using 0.45-µm filters, aliquoted as 500-µL vials, and stored at –20°C. Hybridization buffer should be always used as a 7:3 ratio of hybridization buffer and any other solution, such as water or painting probe, respectively.

12. We purchase whole-chromosome, chromosome-arm, or centromere painting probes from the American Laboratory Technologies and Vysis.

13. We strongly recommend the HYBrite denaturation/hybridization unit for the automated denaturation and hybridization of the chromosomes. It works as a hot plate for the microscope slides. It can be programmed to different temperatures and times, as can PCR machines. Otherwise, chromosomes should be denatured manually.

14. pH is adjusted by 1 N citric acid.

15. Nonfat dry milk is dissolved in solution III, and sterilized using a 0.45-µm filter.

16. We generally use anti-DIG-FITC (Roche, Applied Science) for the detection of probe hybridization and anti-biotin-Texas Red (Rockland Immunochemicals, Inc.) for the detection of biotin-labeled chromosome painting probes.

17. Established cell cultures should be subcultured the day before metaphase chromosome preparation, because it is important to obtain actively proliferating cells. Generally five to six mitotic cells per view are enough to proceed.

18. Vinblastine binds to microtubular proteins of the mitotic spindle, leading to

crystallization of the microtubule and mitotic arrest. Some protocols use colcemid, a colchicine analog, to a final concentration of 0.1 μg/mL for the same purpose. Vinblastine is known to be more effective and gentler on mitotic arrest.

19. Hypotonic treatment causes swelling of the cells. The optimal time of KCl treatment varies from cell type to cell type and must be determined empirically. But we recommend 4 min for the human lymphoblastoid cells and 15 min for the mouse–human hybrid cells.

20. Fixed cells can be kept at –20°C for a maximum of 1 yr. Before they are used again, a freshly prepared fixative solution is added to the cells to a volume of 10 mL and cells are centrifuged for 5 min at 400g and dissolved in an appropriate volume of fixative according to the cell density. According to our protocol, about 50 μL of the fixative results in an adequate number of cell spreads when 5–10 μL of this solution is dropped onto the microscope slides.

21. After dropping the cells onto microscope slides, cell density, the number of metaphase spreads, and the quality of chromosome preparation should be examined under the microscope. Chromosomes should be dark gray when viewed under phase contrast. If the cell number is too low, the cell solution volume to be dropped can be increased or the cells can be centrifuged and dissolved in less fixative solution. If the cell number is too high, cells can be further diluted with fixative solution. To a certain degree, this can also be a solution if the number of metaphase spreads is low. Sometimes, the number of intact cells can be too high and there can be some granules in the cell environment. Repetition of fixative treatment (fixative addition and centrifugation) can solve the problem. Duration of slide drying is also critical. It should not be too fast or too slow. To dry them, blowing gently can be helpful. Another widely used strategy is to drop the cells on steam-warmed slides. There are many reported ways of chromosome slide preparation. It is best to try different strategies and use the most efficient one.

22. Slides can be used for hybridization the same day as they are made. However, they can be stored several weeks in a dark, clean environment at room temperature or frozen at –80°C for more than 1 yr. Once thawed, the slides should not be frozen again.

23. Precipitated, labeled probes can be kept at –20°C for several years.

24. Manufacturers' suggested amounts of the chromosome painting probes are added to the precipitated labeled probe.

25. Small air bubbles can be squeezed out from the sides by gentle pressing.

26. If chromosomes are denatured manually, then the slides can be incubated in a denaturing solution (70% [v/v] deionized formamide, 2X SSC, 0.1 mM EDTA, pH 7.0) in a fume hood in a 70°C water bath for 2 min. They are quickly dipped in ice-cold 2X SSC and kept in ice-cold 70% ethanol for 1 min. Slides are dehydrated through ethanol series of 70, 85, and 100% for 1 min each and air-dried (not longer than 10 min). The probe is added, and slides are covered by a cover slip and left to incubate in a moist environment at 37°C overnight.

27. A glass plate can be placed on ice in a container, and denatured chromosome

slides can be placed on it.

28. A humid environment is necessary to avoid evaporation and slide drying. Paper towels are soaked in water and placed on the empty spaces of HYBrite. If hybridization is carried out in an incubator, a moist environment can be created in a conveniently sized container or chamber with a lid. Slides are lined up on the bottom of container (not on top of one another). Soaked towels are folded up into rolls and placed on the empty spaces, and the container covered with the lid. For use with light-sensitive reagents, the moist chamber is wrapped with aluminum foil.

29. Wash stringency (temperature and salt concentration) can be adjusted for the optimum hybridization results.

30. Antibody dilution should be optimized for each new batch of antibody. As a reference, we use 1:100 dilution of Anti-DIG-FITC and 1:25 dilution of anti-biotin-Texas Red.

Acknowledgments

The authors would like to thank Dr. Olga B. Chernova for her technical advice and guidance throughout the FISH experiments and fluorescence microscopy. This work was supported by the National Institutes of Health (NIH) grants R01 HL65630, R01 HL66251, and P50 HL77107, and an American Heart Association Established Investigator award (to Q.W.).

References

1. Buckle, V. J. and Keraney L. (1994) New methods in cytogenetics. *Curr. Opin. Genet. Dev.* **4,** 374–382.

2. Weier, H. U., Wang, M., Mullikin, J. C., et al. (1995) Quantitative DNA fiber mapping. *Hum. Mol. Genet.* **4,** 1903–1910.

3. Lengauer, C., Green, E. D., and Cremer, T. (1992) Fluorescence in situ hybridization of YAC clones after Alu-PCR amplification. *Genomics* **13,** 826–828.

4. Vooijs, M., Yu, L. C., Tkachuk, D., Pinkel, D., Johnson, D., and Gray, J. W. (1993) Libraries for each human chromosome, constructed from sorter-enriched chromosomes by using linker-adaptor PCR. *Am. J. Hum. Genet.* **52,** 586–597.

5. Lichter, P., Cremer, T., Bordern, J, Manuelidis, L., and Ward, D. C. (1988) Delineation of individual human chromosomes in metaphase and interphase cells by in situ suppression hybridization using chromosome specific library probes. *Hum. Genet.* **80,** 224–234.

6. Rigby, P. W. J., Dieckmann, M., Rhodes, C., and Berg, P. (1977) Labeling deoxyribonucleic acid to high specific activity in vitro by nick translation with DNA polymerase I. *J. Mol. Biol.* **113,** 237–241.

7. Schröck, E., du Manoir, S., Veldman, T., et al. (1996) Multicolor spectral karyotyping of human chromosomes. *Science* **273,** 494–497.

8. Wang, Q., Timur, A. A., Szafranski, P., et al. (2001) Identification and molecular characterization of de novo translocation t(8;14)(q22.3;q13) associated with a vascular and tissue overgrowth syndrome. *Cytogenet. Cell Genet.* **95,** 183–188.

9. Timur, A. A., Sadgephour, A., Graf, M., et al. (2004) Identification and molecular

characterization of a *de novo* supernumerary ring chromosome 18 in a patient with Klippel-Trenaunay syndrome. *Ann. Hum. Genet.* **68,** 353–361.

3

Comparative Genomic Hybridization by Microarray for the Detection of Cytogenetic Imbalance

Malgorzata Jarmuz, Blake C. Ballif, Catherine D. Kashork, Aaron P. Theisen, Bassem A. Bejjani, and Lisa G. Shaffer

Summary

Chromosomal abnormalities often result in the improper dosage of genes in a particular chromosome or chromosome segment, which may cause specific and complex clinical phenotypes. Comparative genomic hybridization by microarray (array CGH) is a high-throughput and high-resolution method for the detection of microscopic and submicroscopic chromosome abnormalities, some of which may not be detectable by conventional cytogenetic techniques. In addition, with the human genome sequenced and publicly available, array CGH allows for the direct correlation between chromosomal anomalies and genomic sequence. Properly constructed, microarrays have the potential to be a valuable tool for the detection of chromosomal abnormalities in cancer and genetic disease.

Key Words: Array CGH; microarray; comparative genomic hybridization; chromosomal abnormalities; cytogenetics; molecular cytogenetics; DNA copy number.

1. Introduction

Comparative genomic hybridization by microarray (array CGH) is a high-throughput, high-resolution method that allows for the detection of genome-wide and chromosome-specific copy number imbalances. Array CGH was developed to increase the resolution of conventional CGH (*1,2*), in which two differentially labeled genomes, a test and control, are competitively hybridized to metaphase chromosomes. Array CGH replaces the metaphase chromosomes with target DNA segments that have been immobilized on a glass slide in an ordered fashion (*see* **Note 1**). The targets may be complementary DNA (cDNA), oligonucleotides, or large-insert genomic clones (e.g., bacterial artificial chromosomes [BACs]). Two genomic DNAs, a test and reference, are

From: *Methods in Molecular Medicine, Vol. 128: Cardiovascular Disease; Methods and Protocols; Volume 1*
Edited by: Q. Wang © Humana Press Inc., Totowa, NJ

then fluorescently labeled and competitively hybridized to the arrayed targets. Following hybridization, imaging systems quantify and compare the hybridization ratios between the test and control DNAs. Because the targets for analysis are orders of magnitude smaller than metaphase chromosomes or chromosomal segments, the resolution of array CGH is substantially increased over that of conventional CGH: although the resolution of conventional CGH on metaphase chromosomes is limited to 3–5 Mb *(3–5)*, only the size of the clones and the distance between them is a limiting factor in the resolution of array CGH. In addition, compared with fluorescence *in situ* hybridization (FISH), in which only a single target may be interrogated at a time, hundreds or thousands of clones can be analyzed simultaneously with array CGH. Array CGH can be used for clinical diagnosis, but the microarray for this purpose must be constructed with some precautions *(6)*. It must be reliable, allow accurate detection of the chromosomal abnormalities, and provide interpretable results. The first step in the development of a clinical microarray is choosing the regions of interest based on clinical significance. The genomic/chromosomal location of selected clones should be verified by FISH prior to immobilizing on the array *(6)*. Clones that map to multiple locations cannot be used for array CGH, as they may provide erroneous results allowing for misinterpretation of the clinical diagnosis. However, if constructed carefully, microarrays are important diagnostic tools for the detection of chromosomal abnormalities.

2. Materials

2.1. Preparation of Aminosilane-Coated Slides

1. 3-Aminopropyltrimethoxysilane (Sigma).
2. Acetone, high-performance liquid chromatography (HPLC)-grade.
3. NaOH.
4. Ethanol.
5. Low-autofluorescence slide (VWR International, West Chester, PA).
6. Staining jars with slide holders.

2.2. Microarray Construction

1. DNA extracted and purified from selected genomic clones.
2. RPM SPIN Midi kit (Q-BIO gene, Carlsbad, CA).
3. 3 *M* Sodium acetate, pH 5.2.
4. Isopropanol.
5. Sterile water.
6. Dimethylsulfoxide (DMSO) with nitrocellulose: dissolve 1.85 g nitrocellulose in 50 mL DMSO (can be stored in room temperature wrapped in aluminum foil); solution for printing: add 1 µL DMSO/nitrocellulose solution to 99 µL DMSO

(when stored in refrigeration, the solution may contain a precipitate. Once warmed, the precipitate will go into solution) *(7)*.

7. 95% Ethanol.
8. 70% Ethanol.
9. 10% Bovine serum albumin fraction V (Sigma).
10. Salmon sperm DNA (Invitrogen).
11. Sonicator.
12. Microarrayer.
13. 384-Well plates.

2.3. Probe Preparation

1. Genomic DNA from lymphoblastoid cell lines, peripheral blood or tissue from subject (*see* **Note 2**).
2. Genomic DNA from phenotypically normal male and female references.
3. *Dpn II* (New England Biolabs).
4. Phenol/chloroform (Amresco).
5. Chloroform (Amresco).
6. 3 *M* Sodium acetate (NaAc), pH 5.2.
7. Isopropanol.
8. Bio Prime DNA labeling system (Invitrogen).
9. Cyanine3 (Cy3-dUTP or Cy3-dCTP) (Perkin Elmer).
10. Cyanine5 (Cy5-dUTP or Cy5-dCTP) (Perkin Elmer).
11. DNA Triphosphate set (Roche).
12. Microcon filter units (Millipore).
13. Human Cot-1 DNA (Invitrogen).
14. 5 *M* NaCl (Sigma).
15. ULTRAhyb (Ambion).

2.4. Hybridization

1. Cover slip.
2. Incubation chamber (Corning Incorporated Life Sciences).
3. Microarray.
4. Probes (labeled genomic DNA from subject and reference).
5. Deionized formamide (VWR).
6. 20X SSC (VWR).
7. Rubber cement.

2.5. Postwashes

1. Phosphate-buffered saline (PBS).
2. 20X SSC: 175.3 g NaCl, 88.2 g Na citrate.
3. Deionized formamide (VWR).
4. Sodium dodecyl sulfate (SDS).

2.6. Microarray Analysis

1. Dual-laser scanner (e.g., GenePix 4000B, Axon Instruments).
2. Imaging software (e.g., GenePix Pro 5.0 and Acuity, Axon Instruments).

3. Methods

3.1. Preparation of Aminosilane-Coated Slides (7)

1. Fill the slide holder with 19 clean (*see* **Note 3**) slides. Place the slides in holder in a zig-zag pattern.
2. Prepare wash solution: dissolve 30 g of NaOH pellets in 120 mL deionized water and add 180 mL of ethanol (200 mL wash solution per slide jar). Because NaOH may oxidize, prepare a fresh solution for every experiment. **Note:** NaOH is poisonous, corrosive, and can cause severe burns.
3. Place the holder into the NaOH solution and shake gently for at least 2 h. To avoid contamination with dust, keep the slides submerged.
4. Place the slide holder in a large container and rinse the slides under deionized water at least 3 min. Keep the slides submerged in water.
5. Place jars in absolute ETOH for 3 min, spin-dry for 3 min at 1400 rpm, then bake at 80°C for 15 min.
6. Prepare the eight slide containers in a fume hood as follows:

   Jar 1: 70% acetone (HPLC grade).
   Jar 2: coating solution: add 200 mL of aminosilane to 200 mL HPLC-grade acetone. Mix solution with a glass rod.
   Jar 3: 70% acetone.
   Jar 5: 70% acetone.
   Jar 6: 70% acetone.
   Jar 7: 70% acetone.
   Jar 8: 95% ethanol.

7. Place the slide rack containing slides into jar 1 to remove water. Let it sit for approx 30 s while gently pulling it up and down out of the jar.
8. Submerge the slide rack into jar 2. Shake gently for 2 min.
9. Wash slides in 70% acetone in each of the next five jars for 2 min each.
10. Move the rack with slides to jar 8 with 95% ethanol. The slides can be kept submerged in ethanol before drying.
11. Spin slides at 380*g* for 1 min (prepare two racks of coated slides for simultaneous centrifugation for convenience).
12. Age the coated slides in their glass racks for 3 d at 80°C prior to storing.
13. Store the slides in a slide box until use.

3.2. Microarray Construction

1. Selected clones (BACs, P1 artificial chromosomes [PACs], yeast artificial chromosomes [YACs], cosmids, fosmids, plasmids, and so on) are grown in LB medium with appropriate antibiotic. The DNA insert is extracted using commercially available midi kits.

2. Sonicate *(7)* 5 µg of DNA insert to a final size between 500 bp and 20 kb.
   a. Place 5 µg of DNA insert in 200 µL deionized water in 1.5-mL tube. Place the tube containing DNA on the shaker for 10 min at 1000 rpm. Next, briefly spin the DNA to the bottom of the tube.
   b. Prepare the sonicator: rinse the sonicator probe thoroughly with water. Fill the falcon 2053 (12 × 75 mm) tube with water and sonicate under the same conditions as for a DNA sample (20% power, cycle 1, no. seconds of effective sonication time). Dry the probe using paper tissue. Wear ear protection.
   c. Place the sonicator probe as deep as possible into the solution of DNA, being sure not to touch the tube. Start sonication by pressing the start button on the timer for at least 1 s. Clean the sonicator probe thoroughly and unplug the sonicator.
   d. After sonication, check size of DNA insert using 2 µL of DNA on 1% agarose mini gel, with the smallest possible width of combs. Use λ-*Hin*dIII and 123-bp ladder as size markers. If there is a large band at the top of the gel, the DNA should be resonicated, using the same settings as before or a shorter time (*see* **Note 4**).
3. Precipitate extracted DNA insert with 3 *M* of NaAc (1:8 of the total volume) and isopropanol (1:1 vol). Mix well.
4. Leave at –0°C 1 h or at –20°C overnight.
5. Centrifuge at 14,000–16,000*g* for 8 min.
6. Wash DNA pellet with 70% ethanol.
7. Centrifuge at 14,000–16,000*g* for 8 min and remove supernatant. Let DNA pellet dry 10–15 min.
8. Hydrate DNA pellet with 8 µL of sterile water.
9. Add 50% dimethylsulfoxide (DMSO) with nitrocellulose before printing slides.
10. Place selected DNA clones in 384-well plate and print on the aminosilane-coated slides using a microarray printer at 30% humidity and temperature of 24°C.
11. Bake the printed slides at 80°C from 4 h to overnight and wash with 80°C Millipure water for 2 min and ice-cold 95% ethanol for 1 min.
12. Block the slide under a cover slip with 10% bovine serum albumin fraction V and 20 µg salmon sperm DNA in a humid chamber at 45°C for 2 h.
13. Denature the slide by washing in 80°C Millipore water for 2 min, dehydrate with ice-cold 95% ethanol for 1 min, and store in a dessicator.

3.3. Genomic DNA Label Preparation

1. Digest 12.5 µg of genomic DNAs separately from subject and reference with *Dpn*II (*see* **Note 5**).
2. Stop the digest and precipitate the digest reaction with an equal volume of phenol/chloroform. Vortex and transfer top phase to a clean tube. Precipitate the reaction again with an equal volume of chloroform. Vortex and transfer top phase to a clean tube.
3. Reprecipitate digested DNA with 1:8 vol of NaAc 3 *M* pH 5.2 and 1:1 vol isopropanol.

4. Leave at –70°C 1 h or at –20°C overnight.
5. Centrifuge at 14,000–16,000g for 8 min.
6. Wash DNA pellet with 70% ethanol.
7. Centrifuge at 14,000–16,000g for 8 min and remove supernatant. Let DNA pellet dry for 10–15 min.
8. Resuspend DNA in 20 μL sterile water.
9. Place 1 μL DNA in a microcentrifuge tube with 11 μL of sterile Millipore water (there should be two label tubes for the patient and two label tubes for the control).
10. Add 10 μL of 2.5X random primer solution (included in kit) to each sample. Incubate at 95°C in water bath for 5 min. Immediately cool on ice for 5 min.
11. Add on ice to each tube: two tubes of reference DNA for two different dyes and two tubes of subject DNA for two different dyes. Work in the dark.

	DNAs labeled with Cy3		DNAs labeled with Cy5	
	Subject	Reference	Subject	Reference
10X nucleotide mix	1.25 μL	1.25 μL	1.25 μL	1.25 μL
Cy3-dCTP	0.75 μL	0.75 μL	–	–
Cy5-dCTP	–	–	0.75 μL	0.75 μL
Exo-KlenovFragment	1 μL	1 μL	1 μL	1 μL

12. Mix and centrifuge just enough to bring the solution into the bottom of the tube. Incubate 37°C for 2 h.
13. Add 2.5 μL stop buffer (from kit) to each tube and place on ice.
14. Purify probes with Microcon filter units.
15. Combine 500 ng of subject's DNA, labeled with Cy3 (green), with an equal concentration of reverse-sex reference DNA labeled with Cy5 (red). In a second tube, combine oppositely labeled (Cy5) subject DNA with an equal amount of oppositely labeled (Cy3) reverse-sex reference DNA.
16. Add 50 μg of Cot1-DNA and reprecipitate.
17. Hydrate the probes with 15.5 μL ULTRAhyb.

3.4. Hybridization

1. Perform all steps in the dark.
2. Denature labeled genomic DNA probes at 72°C for 5 min.
3. Preanneal immediately at 37°C for 1 h (*see* **Note 6**).
4. Place the probe onto a microarray and cover with a 22 × 22 mm cover slip. Be sure that there are no bubbles under the cover slip (*see* **Note 7**).
5. Hybridize at 37°C in an incubation chamber with shaking for 14–16 h.

3.5. Posthybridization Washes

1. Perform all steps in the dark.

2. Remove the cover slip by soaking in 1X PBS.
3. Wash the microarrays with 50% formamide, 2X SSC, 0.1% SDS at 45°C 20 min and 1X PBS for 20 min at room temperature.
4. Rinse in 0.2X SSC, followed by Millipore water. Dry immediately.

3.6. Microarray Analysis

The analysis of array CGH is performed in three steps. In the first step, the images are acquired using a dual-laser scanner. Two simultaneous scans of each array at two differential wavelengths (635 and 532 nm) are required. The next step is the quantification of fluorescence intensity. The individual spots are analyzed with imaging software. The clones may be spotted on the microarray three to four times for assessing result reproducibility. The average ratios of these spots for each subject are analyzed with software. The background noise is subtracted and the ratio of fluorescence intensities derived from hybridized test and reference DNA are calculated and normalized by the ratios measured from reference spots on the same slide. The results are converted to $\log_2$ scale and plotted in an interpretable format (**Fig. 1**). Establishing the specificity of the system and setting a baseline threshold are performed by experimental results of normal variation observed after cohybridization of two normal reference DNAs to the microarray.

4. Notes

1. In microarray terminology, the term "target" refers to the DNA bounded to the glass slides, and the term "probe" defines the labeled genomic DNA.
2. The purity and quality of genomic DNA is very important to obtain high-quality results. Low-quality DNA can result in high background and low signal intensity on the microarray.
3. Dirty slides can cause high levels of background and should be discarded.
4. It is important not to start precipitation before obtaining the results from the agarose gel. The sizes of BAC DNA should be 500 bp to 20 kb. Sonication reduces the size of BAC DNA significantly, thus reducing the viscosity of the printing solutions; this helps in reliably depositing the clone DNA on the solid support (glass slide).
5. Digestion of gemomic DNA by restriction enzymes is very important for labeling efficiency. Decreasing the average fragment size may increase labeling efficiency, but if the fragments are too small, the hybridization and subsequent results may be affected.
6. Preannealing the probes allows for sufficient blocking of repetitive elements.
7. The microarray must not dry during any hybridization step; ensure that the hybridization chamber remains humidified to prevent evaporation of the probe or blocking mixture. Otherwise, the results will be unusable.

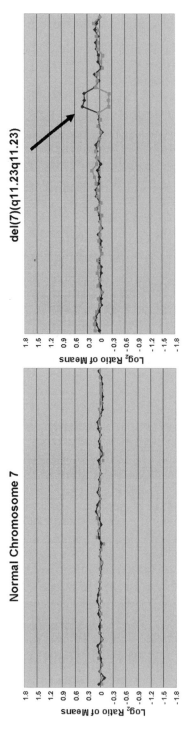

Fig. 1. Detection of a deletion in the Williams syndrome region using a targeted array. Each clone on the plot is arranged along the x-axis according to its location on the chromosome, with the most distal/telomeric short-arm clones on the left and the most distal/telomeric long-arm clones on the right. The dark blue line represents the control:patient fluorescence intensity ratios for each clone, whereas the pink line represents the fluorescence intensity ratios obtained from a second hybridization in which the dyes have been reversed (patient:control). On the left is a plot for a normal chromosome 7. On the right is a plot for an individual with a del (7) (q11.23q11.23). The normal chromosome 7 plot shows a ratio of 0 on a log$_2$ scale for all clones. The plot showing the deletion of 7q11.23 shows a significant deviation from 0 for the three clones that have a single-copy loss in the individual. The proximal and distal flanking clones were not deleted.

References

1. Pinkel, D., Segraves, R., Sudar D., et al. (1998) High resolution analysis of DNA copy number variation using comparative genomic hybridization to microarrays. *Nat. Genet.* **20,** 207–211.
2. Solinas-Toldo, S., Lampel, S., Stilgenbauer, S., et al. (1997) Matrix-based comparative genomic hybridization: biochips to screen for genomic imbalances. *Genes Chromosomes Cancer* **20,** 399–407.
3. Kallioniemi, A., Kallioniemi, O. P., Sudar, D., et al. (1992) Comparative genomic hybridization for molecular cytogenetic analysis of solid tumors. *Science* **258,** 818-821.
4. Kallioniemi O. P., Kallioniemi A., Sudar D., et al. (1993) Comparative genomic hybridization: a rapid new method for detecting and mapping DNA amplification in tumors. *Semin. Cancer Biol.* **4,** 41-46.
5. Kirchhoff, M., Gerdes, T., Maahr, J., et al. (1999) Deletions below 10 megabasepairs are detected in comparative genomic hybridization by standard reference intervals. *Genes Chromosomes Cancer* **25,** 410–413.
6. Bejjani, B. A., Saleki, R., Ballif, B. C., et al. (2005) Use of targeted array-based CGH for the clinical diagnosis of chromosomal imbalance: is less more? *Am. J. Med. Genet. A.* **134,** 259–267.
7. Buckley, P. G., Mantripragada, K. K., Benetkiewicz, M., et al. (2002) A full-coverage, high-resolution human chromosome 22 genomic microarray for clinical and research applications. *Hum. Mol. Genet.* **11,** 3221–3219.

4

Construction of Somatic Cell Hybrid Lines

*Fusion of Mouse Thymidine Kinase-Deficient 3T3 Fibroblasts
and Human Lymphoblastoid Cells*

Ayse Anil Timur and Qing K. Wang

Summary

Somatic cell hybrids are generated by fusion of two different parental cells. This technology has been used extensively in the production of monoclonal antibodies and has made significant contributions to the field of human genetics through its applications in gene expression, gene mapping, and positional cloning of human disease genes. In our laboratory, we have employed this technique in the positional cloning of several genes for human diseases associated with cytogenetic abnormalities (chromosomal disorders), including translocations. Somatic cell hybrids are constructed by fusing mouse thymidine kinase-deficient 3T3 fibroblasts with human lymphoblastoid cells, as a result of which specific hybrid cells containing only cytogenetically abnormal human chromosomes involved in a chromosomal disorder can be successfully isolated and cloned. These hybrid cells serve as an excellent tool with which to define the exact chromosomal breakpoints involved in a cytogenetic abnormality and to identify genes at the breakpoints.

Key Words: Somatic cell hybrids; positional cloning; polyethylene glycol; PEG; cell fusion; HAT selection; ring cloning; subcloning.

1. Introduction

Cultured somatic cells can be induced to fuse together to form combined cells with two nuclei called heterokaryons, which eventually proceed to mitosis and form hybrid cells with one fused nucleus. Somatic cell hybrids can be produced from two different species such as rodents and humans (interspecific hybrids) or two different cells from the same species (intraspecific hybrids). For unknown reasons, as rodent–human hybrid cells proliferate, they lose human chromosomes randomly, which results in hybrid cell lines, each of them

From: *Methods in Molecular Medicine, Vol. 128: Cardiovascular Disease; Methods and Protocols; Volume 1*
Edited by: Q. Wang © Humana Press Inc., Totowa, NJ

containing a variety of one or a few human chromosomes. The most widespread use of somatic cell hybrids is the formation of hybridomas for monoclonal antibody production *(1)*. They have also been used in genetic complementation studies. Probably the most significant uses of somatic cell hybrids are the chromosomal mapping of genes or markers *(2)* and the positional cloning of the disease genes for human diseases associated with a cytogenetic abnormalities such as translocations, deletions, duplications, inversions, or other defects *(3,4)*.

The construction of somatic hybrid cell lines involves cell fusion, selection, isolation, propagation, and characterization of hybrids. Cell fusions were initially carried out using UV-inactivated Sendai virus, which has been replaced by an easier, quicker, and more efficient technique using polyethylene glycol (PEG) *(5)*. After fusion, a selection system is necessary to eliminate the cells that cannot yield hybrids. Hypoxanthine, aminopterin, thymidine (HAT) selection is the most commonly used system *(6)*. Aminopterin blocks the main pathway of DNA synthesis. However, if cells are supplied with hypoxanthine and thymidine, they can synthesize DNA via a salvage pathway using hypoxanthine phosphoribosyl transferase (HPRT) and thymidine kinase (TK). Thus, normal cells grow quite well in HAT-supplied media. But, cells deficient in HPRT or TK cannot survive in the presence of HAT and die, which is the basis of HAT selection. There are also other selection agents such as quabain and G418 *(7,8)*.

Because of different chromosomal content, hybrid cell lines have different growth rates. Individual hybrid clones should be isolated to prevent rapidly growing hybrid clones from dominating the culture. Ring cloning is a widely used isolation technique for the hybrids of anchorage-dependent, monolayer cells. Single-cell isolation cloning can also be carried out under a microscope *(9)*. The isolated colonies are then expanded.

Hybrid cell lines should be characterized for their chromosome content as quickly as possible to minimize the labor and time involved in the culturing of hybrid cells that do not contain the chromosome(s) of interest. Chromosome staining techniques, fluorescence *in situ* hybridization (FISH), and PCR for the presence of certain genetic markers, which are known to reside on the chromosome(s) of interest, are the techniques used in the characterization of hybrid cells *(9)*. Even an isolated, cloned hybrid cell line is often a mixture of cells containing subgroups of the main chromosome content and can be subcloned to isolate new cell lines that lose additional chromosomes. Single human chromosomes can also be transferred into a recipient cell using microcell-mediated chromosome transfer (MMCT) called microcell fusion *(10)*.

In our laboratory, somatic cell hybrids were generated through the cell fusions of mouse TK-deficient 3T3 fibroblasts and human lymphoblastoid cells for the positional cloning of several human disease genes. Human lymphoblastoid cells were prepared from several patients carrying a chromosomal translocation. Hybrid cell lines containing each derivative chromosome without their normal chromosome homolog were successfully characterized and maintained. PCR analysis of sequence-tagged sites (STSs) was then used to examine whether each STS is present or absent on the derivative chromosome from the hybrid cell. The chromosome breakpoint is then defined between one STS showing the presence on the derivative chromosome and a neighbor STS showing the absence. The gene or genes disrupted by the breakpoint or located close to the breakpoint are considered as the candidate gene(s) for the disease, and are further characterized.

2. Materials
2.1. Cell Fusion

1. Mouse TK-deficient 3T3 and human lymphoblastoid cell cultures (*see* **Note 1**).
2. Dulbecco's modified Eagle's medium (DMEM) supplemented with 10% fetal bovine serum (FBS) and 1X antibiotic-antimycotic solution (Gibco BRL) (*see* **Note 2**).
3. Serum-free DMEM.
4. 50% (w/v) PEG 1000 (*see* **Note 3**).
5. Phosphate-buffered saline (PBS) solution (*see* **Note 4**).
6. 50X HAT supplement (Sigma or Invitrogen GIBCO Cell Culture Systems) 5 mM sodium hypoxanthine, 20 μM aminopterin, 0.8 mM thymidine (*see* **Note 5**).
7. 15-mL conical-bottom plastic tubes.
8. 100-mm tissue-culture plates.

2.2. Hybrid Isolation by Ring Cloning

1. PBS.
2. Sterile vacuum grease (*see* **Note 6**).
3. Trypsin/EDTA solution: 5% (w/v) trypsin, 2% (w/v) EDTA.
4. DMEM supplemented with 10% FBS and 1X antibiotic-antimycotic solution (Gibco BRL).
5. Sterile cloning rings (*see* **Note 7**).
6. 96-, 24-, and 6-Well, and 100-mm, tissue-culture plates.

2.3. Subcloning of Hybrids

1. DMEM supplemented with 10% FBS and 1X antibiotic-antimycotic solution (Gibco BRL).
2. 96-Well microtiter plate.

2.4. DNA Isolation for Characterization of Hybrids by PCR

1. Cell lysis buffer: 10 mM Tris-HCl, pH 8.3, 1.25 mM Mg Cl$_2$, 50 mM KCl, 0.01% gelatin, 0.45% Tween-20, 0.45% NP 40. Autoclave and store at room temperature (*see* **Note 8**).

2. Proteinase K.
3. 1.5-mL Eppendorf tube.

3. Methods

All cell media with or without serum, PBS, trypsin/EDTA, and 50% PEG, are prewarmed to 37°C, and all cell culture incubations are performed in a humidified 37°C, 10% CO_2 incubator.

3.1. Cell Fusion

1. Both human lymphoblastoid and mouse TK-deficient 3T3 cell lines are harvested separately and washed once with PBS.
2. 5×10^6 cells from each parent cell line are mixed in a 15-mL conical-bottom plastic tube and cosedimented by centrifuging for 5 min at 400g.
3. The mixture of cells is washed three times with 10 mL of PBS to remove serum completely.
4. After the final wash, liquid is aspirated, but 20 µL is left in the tube. Pellet is loosened by flicking tube gently.
5. 0.5 mL of 50% PEG is added to the pellet and tube is flicked gently for 1 min (*see* **Note 9**).
6. 10 mL of serum-free medium is added and tube is inverted gently. The tube is centrifuged for 5 min at 400g.
7. Serum-free medium washing (**step 6**) is repeated twice.
8. Pellet is resuspended in 6 mL of DMEM with serum and 1 mL of cell suspension is distributed into 100-mm tissue culture plates containing 9 mL of DMEM and 1X HAT selective reagent (*see* **Notes 10** and **11**).
9. Plates are incubated and the medium is refreshed after 3–4 d.

3.2. Colony Isolation by Ring Cloning

1. Individual hybrid colonies are circled and numbered with a waterproof marker pen from the undersides of the plates (*see* **Note 12**).
2. Cells are washed once with 10 mL of PBS and all solutions are aspirated.
3. One end of a sterile cloning ring is coated with sterile vacuum grease by dipping it in a grease-containing Petri dish using a pair of sterile forceps. Grease is flattened as a thin layer and excess is removed by using a sterile pipet tip. Using forceps, cloning ring is placed over a selected colony, which was marked previously on bottom of a dish (*see* **Note 13**).
4. When all targeted colonies are recovered, two to three drops of trypsin/EDTA are added to each recovered colony and the plate is left until cells begin to detach.
5. 30 µL of DMEM with 10% serum is added to each trypsinized colony, and the entire contents of the ring are transferred to a 96-well plate (*see* **Note 14**).
6. The required amount of DMEM with serum and 1X HAT are added to the empty rings and whole plate. Plates are returned to the incubator until new colonies appear (*see* **Note 15**).

7. Picked colonies are expanded, characterized, and frozen (*see* **Note 16**).

3.3. Subcloning of the Hybrid Clones

1. Cloned hybrid cells are counted and diluted to 5 cells/mL of medium with serum and 1X HAT, and 0.2 mL of this solution is dispensed into each well of a 96-well plate so that an average of one cell is added to the each well. The plate is incubated.
2. The wells containing single colonies are expanded, characterized, and frozen (*see* **Note 17**).

3.4. DNA Isolation From Hybrid Clones

1. Hybrid cells are grown to confluence (*see* **Note 18**).
2. Cells are trypsinized and recovered by centrifugation.
3. The cell pellet is resuspended in 25 µL of cell lysis buffer and transferred into a 1.5-mL Eppendorf tube.
4. Proteinase K is added to a final concentration of 1 mg/mL and the mixture is incubated for 1 h at 55°C.
5. Proteinase K is heat inactivated at 95°C for 10 min.
6. The solution is microfuged for 30 s at the maximum speed.
7. 2–3 µL of the clarified supernatant is used for PCR analysis (*see* **Note 19**).

4. Notes

1. Mouse TK-deficient 3T3 fibroblasts are anchorage-dependent, monolayer cells. Human lymphoblastoid cells are anchorage-independent cells growing in suspension culture. Both cell lines grow very well in DMEM supplemented with 10% serum.
2. For antibiotic-antimycotic, 100X solution is purchased from Invitrogen. It contains 10,000 U/mL penicillin G sodium, 10,000 µg/mL streptomycin sulfate, and 25 µg/mL amphotericin B.
3. PEG is a highly water-soluble polymer of ethylene oxide. It dehydrates cell membranes and causes clustering of membrane proteins that are important for cell fusion. PEG with a molecular weight of 1000–1500 can be used for cell fusion. It is solid at room temperature and heated to 65°C to melt. Then, the required amount is weighed into a glass bottle. Because PEG is light sensitive, it should be stored in a dark bottle or in a bottle wrapped with aluminum foil. It is sterilized by autoclaving. PEG is diluted at a 1:1 ratio with serum-free media at 37°C to prepare 50% working solution. We recommend that 50% PEG be freshly prepared each time and stored at 37°C just prior to cell fusion. PEG does not usually change the pH of the medium significantly; if it does, the medium should be well buffered to retain the original pH.
4. All PBS solutions mentioned here contain 137 mM of NaCl, 2.7 mM of KCl, 8.0 mM of Na_2HPO_4-$7H_2O$, and 1.5 mM of KH_2PO_4.
5. We purchase lyophilized HAT from Sigma. When dissolved in 10 mL of sterile water, it makes a 50X HAT stock solution. It can be also purchased as 50X ready

stock solution form Invitrogen Cell Culture Systems. Aliquots of stock solution are stored at 4°C while in use.

6. Vacuum grease is placed in a glass Petri dish, wrapped with foil, and sterilized by autoclaving.

7. Cloning rings are glass cylinders of varying diameter. It is convenient to have cloning rings with different diameters to cover different sizes of colonies. They can be purchased from Scienceware or BELLCO. But 8 × 8 mm ones are the cloning rings most used to isolate and pick the individual hybrid clones. They are sterilized by autoclaving.

8. Cell lysis solution kept at room temperature can be cloudy by the time it is needed. It will be clear again when it is warmed up. However, a cloudy feature does not affect the efficiency of reaction.

9. PEG is toxic to the cells. Different cells show different sensitivities to PEG. Therefore, PEG exposure time is critical and should be optimized. We recommend 1 min for the mouse TK-deficient 3T3 and human lymphoblastoid cells. PEG and cell mixture should be gently and constantly agitated during the time that the cells are in contact with the fusing agent.

10. It is very important that the fused cells are seeded out at low density, allowing the hybrids to establish their own separate colonies. This also makes the isolation of colonies by ring cloning much easier and lowers the risk of colony cross-contamination.

11. Determining the optimum selective concentration of HAT is critical. This can be tested on recipient mouse TK-deficient 3T3 cells by splitting a confluent 100-mm plate into fifths of medium containing different concentrations of HAT. Generally, after 1 wk of incubation, most of the cells will die. The lowest concentration of HAT that prevents cell growth should be chosen. We suggest the use of 0.5–1X final concentrations of HAT for the selection of somatic cell hybrids of human lymphoblastoid cells and mouse TK-deficient 3T3. Moreover, if chromosomes X and 17 are not of interest in the experiment (HPRT and TK genes are on chromosomes X and 17, respectively), HAT treatment can be stopped after several weeks of fusion.

12. According to our experience, hybrid cells should be visible at the end of 1 wk or at maximum in 2 wk. Individual hybrid colonies are examined under an inverted microscope. They are also visible by the naked eye as small, dense, white-gray areas on an empty plate. Colonies are circled by a marker pen on the underside of plate by holding the plate at a right position or through the microscope, by inserting the pen tip between the underside of the dish and objective lens. A number should also be assigned to each individually selected colony and the number should be tracked during the transfer, expansion, and characterization of the corresponding colony.

13. It is important that the edges of the cylinders are ground smooth to make a good contact with the surface of the plate. The grease level should be evenly distributed through the edges of the cylinder.

14. A new pipet tip and/or pipet should be used for each individual colony in transferring and expanding of the colonies to prevent colony cross-contamination. It should be ensured that the picked colony is successfully transferred to the 96-well plate by checking cells under the microscope.

15. We recommend that 100–150 colonies be picked up during the whole procedure. Plates should be checked every day for colonies that are ready to be picked up. Ten to 15 colonies can be picked up from each 100-mm plate at one time. Therefore, it is important to work fast during the ring cloning procedure to prevent the plate from drying. Transferred rings are still filled with media, because the left cells can produce another colony. At the early stages of the procedure, this can be a backup for a colony that is unsuccessfully transferred or expanded.

16. Colonies are first transferred to 96-well plates and expanded to the next one up in series, e.g., 24- and 6-well, and, finally, 100-mm plates. Other sizes of plates can also be utilized according to colony size and growth. Approximately four to five passages are required to grow cells from a single colony to multiple confluent 100-mm plates. The final 100-mm plates for each colony should be split further for DNA extraction and freezing. It is important that passaging of hybrid cells be kept to a minimum and chromosomal characterization be repeated from time to time, because hybrid cells are not stable and further chromosome losses may occur.

17. Two to five days after the cells are dispensed, each well should be checked under the microscope to identify the wells containing just one cell. Sometimes, two, three, or even more cells with different chromosomal backgrounds can be present in the same well as a result of insufficient dilution. These cells are generally too far from one another in the well and can be distinguished from a recently divided cell.

18. Confluent 100-mm plates are usually the main source of DNA extraction. However, when needed, the same procedure can be applied to 6- and 24-well plates as well.

19. We suggest not using an excess amount of supernatant for PCR, because it can inhibit the reaction.

Acknowledgments

The authors would like to thank Dr. John K. Cowell for his technical advice and guidance and Mary McGraw for her technical support through out the first construction of somatic cell hybrids in our laboratory. This work was supported by the National Institutes of Health (NIH) grants R01 HL65630, R01 HL66251, P50 HL77107, and an American Heart Association Established Investigator award (to Q.W.).

References

1. Kohler, G. and Milstein, C. (1976) Derivation of specific antibody-producing tissue culture and tumor lines by cell fusion. *Eur. J. Immunol.* **6,** 511–519.

2. Kelsell, D. P. and Spurr, N. K. (1997) Gene mapping using somatic cell hybrids. *Methods Mol. Biol.* **68,** 45–52.
3. Sossey-Alaoui, K., Su, G., Malaj, E., Roe, B., and Cowell, J. K. (2002) WAVE3, an acting-polymerization gene, is truncated and inactivated as a result of a constitutional t(1;13)(q21;q12) chromosome translocation in a patient with ganglioneuroblastoma. *Oncogene* **21,** 5967–5974.
4. Tian X. L., Kadaba R., You S. A., et al. (2004) Identification of an angiogenic factor that when mutated causes susceptibility to Klippel-Trenaunay syndrome. *Nature* **427,** 640–645.
5. Boni, L. T. and Hui, S. W. (1987) The mechanism of polyethylene glycol induced fusion in model membranes, in *Cell Fusion,* (Sowers, A. E., ed.), Plenum, NY, pp. 301–330.
6. Littlefield, J. W. (1964) Selection of hybrids from matings of fibroblasts in vitro and their presumed recombinants. *Science* **145,** 709–710.
7. Baker, R. M., Brunette, D. M., Mankovitz, R., et al. (1974) Quabain resistant mutants of mouse and hamster cells in culture. *Cell* **1,** 9–21.
8. Southern, P. J. and Berg, P. (1982) Transformation of mammalian cells to antibiotic resistance with a bacterial gene under control of the SV40 early region promoter. *J. Mol. Appl. Gen.* **1,** 327–341.
9. Cowell, J. K. (1992) Somatic cell hybrids in the analysis of the human genome, in *Human Cytogenetics a Practical Approach,* Volume II, (Rooney, D. E. and Czepulkowski, B. H., eds.), Oxford University Press, NY, pp. 235–252.
10. Ege, T. and Ringertz, N. R. (1974) Preparation of microcells by enucleation of micronucleate cells. *Exp. Cell Res.* **87,** 378–382.

5

LINKAGE Programs

Linkage Analysis for Monogenic Cardiovascular Diseases

Lin Li, Qing K. Wang, and Shaoqi Rao

Summary

Identification of the genes for a human disease provides significant insights into the molecular mechanism underlying the pathogenesis of the disease. A human disease gene can be identified by its chromosomal location (positional cloning). Linkage analysis is a key step in positional cloning. For monogenic disorders with a known inheritance pattern, model-based linkage analysis is effective in mapping the disease location. Therefore, model-based linkage analysis can provide a powerful tool to positional cloning of some specific molecular determinants that co-segregate with disease phenotypes in the isolated samples (e.g., large and multiplex impaired pedigrees). This chapter describes model-based human genetic linkage analysis as implemented in the LINKAGE computer package. First, we introduce the basic concepts and principles for genetic analysis of monogenic disorders. Then, we demonstrate the usages of the programs by analyzing several examples of hypothetical pedigrees with the inheritance modes of autosomal-dominant, autosomal-recessive, and genetic heterogeneity.

Key Words: Linkage; gene; positional cloning; cardiovascular disease; autosomal-dominant; autosomal-recessive; genetic heterogeneity.

1. Genetic Concepts and Background

This section describes the basic genetic concepts and background information to determine the best genetic model and parameters for parametric linkage analysis of a disease.

1.1. Inheritance Models

Prior to linkage analysis, the most likely inheritance model for a disease under study can be determined by pedigree investigations. We describe the segregation characteristics for some common inheritance models.

From: *Methods in Molecular Medicine, Vol. 128: Cardiovascular Disease; Methods and Protocols; Volume 1*
Edited by: Q. Wang © Humana Press Inc., Totowa, NJ

1.1.1. Mendelian Recessive Inheritance

The Mendelian recessive inheritance model describes the segregation pattern of recessive phenotypes inherited in a simple autosomal Mendelian manner. The affected phenotype of a recessive disorder is determined by a recessive allele, and the corresponding unaffected phenotype is determined by a dominant allele. Suppose that a human disease is inherited in a simple Mendelian manner as a recessive phenotype, with affection determined by an allele a and the normal condition by A. Hence, the suffers from this disease are of genotype aa, and people who do not have the disease are either AA or Aa. The pedigree characteristics for a Mendelian recessive disorder are:

1. Generally, the disease appears in the progeny of unaffected parents.
2. The affected progeny includes both males and females.
3. Transmission of the disease phenotype between generations can be interrupted, and its occurrence in a pedigree is "sporadic" and may only observed in the proband *(1)*.
4. Progeny from consanguineous marriages have a significantly high rate of affection.

1.1.2. Mendelian Dominant Inheritance

In Mendelian dominant inheritance, the normal allele is recessive, and the abnormal allele is dominant. Like Mendelian recessive inheritance, the disease locus is on an autosomal chromosome and both sexes are represented among the affected offspring, which rules out the sex-linked recessive inheritance described later. The pedigree characteristics for a Mendelian dominant disorder are:

1. The disease phenotype tends to appear in every generation of the pedigree.
2. Sons and daughters are equally likely to inherit the phenotype from their affected fathers or mothers.

Sometimes, the dominance of the disease allele can be incomplete because heterozygotes (Aa) have a disease symptom between two homozygotes and both alleles can confer different risks to an individual, rendering differential expressions of the disease phenotype among the individuals of three genotypes. This is called "incomplete dominance."

1.1.3. X-Linked Inheritance

A disease gene on the X chromosome can cause a special inheritance pattern, called a parallel pattern of inheritance. The segregation characteristics for an X-lined recessive trait include:

1. All affected individuals are males.
2. Both parents of an affected male have normal phenotypes and the mother is a carrier of the disease allele.

3. A cross-over allelic transmission pattern can be seen, i.e., father to daughters or mother to sons.
4. Because the offspring of an affected father are normal, a disrupted inheritance pattern between generations can be seen.

An X-linked trait or disease can also be inherited in the manner of X-linked dominance, resulting from the dominant role of the disease allele. The pedigree characteristics of X-linked dominance include:

1. There are more affected females than males.
2. Either of the parents of an affected individual must also be affected. An affected mother is a heterozygote, who can transmit the disease allele to either son(s) or daughter(s).
3. Affections can be observed for more than two consecutive generations.

1.2. Lod Score, the Statistic for Model-Based Linkage Analysis

A logarithm of the odds (lod) score, first defined by Morton (1955) *(2)*, is a statistic for log (base 10) of the odds for linkage. For example, a lod score of 3.0, the golden criterion for claiming a genome-wide significant evidence of linkage, corresponds to 1000 times greater likelihood of the alternative hypothesis of linkage between a marker locus and the unobservable disease locus sought for, based on the particular configuration of the phenotypic and genotypic data observed in the studied pedigree, than the null hypothesis of no linkage (i.e., θ, the recombination fraction, is 0.5). A lod score of -2.0 or lower is often used for the exclusion criterion in favor of no linkage, and the lod score values between the two ceilings are inclusive and more data are required to clarify the ambiguity. LINKAGE programs or derivatives can compute both two-point and multipoint lod scores for a pedigree. The two-point linkage analysis is essentially a single-point analysis (regarding the marker data) and the unobserved disease locus is always the other hypothetical point. The mathematic formulation can be described:

$$\text{Lod score or } z(x) = \log_{10}\left[\frac{L\left(\text{Pedigree} \mid \theta = x\right)}{L\left(\text{Pedigree} \mid \theta = 0.50\right)}\right]$$

where L is the likelihood and x takes some value between 0 and 0.49. LINKAGE programs can evaluate the linkage at a variety of recombination fraction values, e.g., 0.001, 0.05, 0.10, 0.20, 0.30, and 0.40, recommended at the Human Gene Mapping VII conference *(3)* to generate a lod score profile for each marker under study.

When marker data are not fully informative, multipoint linkage analysis can be performed to evaluate the linkage evidence at a marker locus or off-marker location by LINKAGE programs by the use of multiple nearby markers altogether. A multipoint analysis attempts to locate the disease gene by testing its most likely position with reference to a fixed map of multiple markers, instead of to a single marker as in two-point linkage analysis. The resulting multipoint lod score quantifies statistical support for the position of a disease gene at a specific location on the established map of markers and can be formulated as follows:

$$\text{Lod score or } z(x) = \log_{10}\left[\frac{L\left(\text{Pedigree} \mid \theta_1, \theta_2, \quad, \theta_n = 0 - 0.49; \theta_{Disease} = x\right)}{L\left(\text{Pedigree} \mid \theta_1, \theta_2, \quad, \theta_n = 0 - 0.49; \theta_{Disease} = 0.50\right)}\right]$$

where x is the location of the disease gene relative to a fixed point on the regional map. Thus, a multipoint lod score is also known as map-specific statistic.

1.3. Type of Loci

The LINKAGE programs can accommodate four types of loci: quantitative trait, codominant, binary factors, and affection status. Binary factors loci can be used to code dominant markers (such as the ABO blood types). Quantitative trait loci describe the disease gene for continuous phenotypes. The genotypes (sometimes called locus phenotypes) at codominant loci are discernible, such as markers of microsatellites and single-nucleotide polymorphisms (SNPs). Affection status loci allow specification of whether pedigree individuals are affected or unaffected with a trait, or at some other points in the spectrum of the affection.

1.4. Liability Classes

The LINKAGE programs allow for assigning genotypic susceptibilities (penetrances) for the disease gene, which corresponds to the specific inheritance models assumed for the studied disease (locus).

1.5. Marker Informatics: Polymorphism Information Content

Polymorphism information content (PIC) is a measure of marker informatics for linkage analysis. It differs from heterogeneity measure by punishing the noninformative case for linkage analysis that heterozygous offspring will not provide useful information if both parents are identically heterozygous. A LINKAGE utility for calculating PIC is available along with the LINKAGE package.

1.6. Genetic Heterogeneity

The term of "genetic heterogeneity" is commonly used to describe the fact that two or more genes act independently to cause an identical clinical trait. In other words, the clinically identical forms of the same disease phenotype can result from different genes. This form of heterogeneity (nonallelic or locus heterogeneity) is distinct from allelic heterogeneity, which refers to multiple effective mutations at the same locus or gene. Locus heterogeneity must be considered when multiple pedigrees are analyzed and the occurrence of hetero-geneity is suspected, especially for genetic analysis of complex human dis-eases. The LINKAGE program HOMOG provides the most commonly used test for heterogeneity based on the admixture likelihood function. The test and heterogeneity lod score computation will be demonstrated using an example in a later section.

2. LINKAGE Programs

The LINKAGE software package covers the most commonly used programs for model-based linkage analysis. The LINKAGE software package is avail-able free of charge from the website at Rockefeller University (http://linkage.rockefeller.edu). We will introduce several programs here and illus-trate their usages in a later section by examples.

2.1. Makeped, a Utility Tool for the LINKAGE Data Format

MAKEPED is a utility tool that converts information on pedigree structure, affection status, and marker genotypes from a simple format, generally called a "pre-MAKEPED" or simply a "pre-" file, into a format appropriate for linkage analysis by the LINKAGE programs. Specifically, MAKEPED performs the following tasks:

1. Checks the pedigree input file for various structural inconsistencies, such as individuals who have only one parent listed, parents of the wrong gender (for instance, both parents listed as females), and individuals unrelated to the pedigree (i.e., unconnected persons).
2. Generates pedigree pointers that direct the LINKAGE program's traversal of the pedigree. For each individual, three pointer fields are added: one field referring to the first offspring, one to the first (or next) paternal sibling, and one to the first (or next) maternal sibling.
3. Adds a proband field. In a pedigree without consanguinity or marriage loops, all entries in the proband field are 0 except for the proband (with a code of 1).

2.2. Unknown for Data Inconsistencies

Before invoking any of the LINKAGE programs, UNKNOWN must be run to perform two main types of data checking:

1. First, it checks the input pedigree file for data inconsistencies (e.g., two parents of the same gender or non-Mendelian segregation of marker alleles) and alerts the user if inconsistencies are found.
2. Second, it deletes any impossible genotypes from consideration in the likelihood calculations for individuals whose disease or marker status is unknown, thereby increasing the speed of the linkage analysis.

UNKNOWN has two output files, ipedfile.dat and speedfil.dat. The ipedfile.dat file is a version of pedfile.dat that has been revised to include the genotypes of untyped individuals that can be inferred with certainty. The speedfil.dat includes a list of possible genotypes for individuals whose genotypes are unknown and cannot be inferred with complete certainty.

2.3. MLINK for Two-Point Lod Score Computation

MLINK computes two-point lod scores for any two loci based on the likelihood of the pedigree under user-specified values of the genetic model parameters or under the null model of no linkage between the two loci, typically, a disease or trait locus and a marker locus. MLINK is the only program that calculates the genetic risks for user-specified individuals.

2.4. Linkmap for Multipoint Lod Score Computation

Linkmap is a LINKAGE program used to compute a multipoint lod score for a pedigree and to determine the most likely location of a marker or disease trait relative to a series of markers whose map is established. Likelihoods of the pedigree data are calculated based on the user-specified order and spacing of two or more markers and the putative location(s) for the trait locus whose position is unknown.

2.5. HOMOG for Heterogeneity Lod Score Computation

The HOMOG programs compute heterogeneity lod scores and can be used to test whether there is significant evidence of genetic heterogeneity among multiple pedigrees. There are several programs that address various scenarios of heterogeneity. HOMOG is used to analyze heterogeneity assuming two family types, either linked or unlinked to a marker locus. HOMOG1 additionally permits gender-specific settings of recombination rates. Other programs (HOMOG2, HOMOG3, and HOMOG4) analyze locus heterogeneity assuming that there are two (or three, or four) family types, and that all families are linked, but to different markers on the same chromosome (*see also* **ref. 4**). HOMOG3R can investigate heterogeneity by allowing three family types, with one type linked to a marker on some chromosome, another type linked to a marker on a different chromosome, and the third type linked to neither marker. HOMOGM allows for heterogeneity incurred by any number of loci (*5*).

3. Implementations by Examples

Two input files are required to performed model-based linkage analysis using the LINKAGE programs: the pedigree and parameter files, which can be made by using a text editor or MAKEPED and PREPLINK, a program designed to generate the parameter file. A pedigree file (pedfile.dat) includes informa-

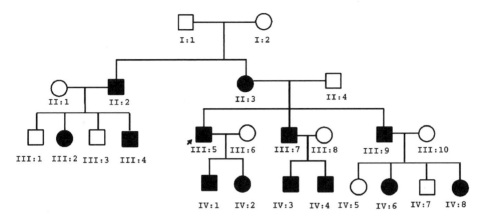

Fig. 1. Pedigree of an artificial family in Example 1. Circles and squares denote female and male family members, respectively. Filled symbols denote affected individuals with the disease, and empty symbols denote those unaffected. The proband is indicated by an arrow.

tion on pedigree relationships, disease affection status, and marker information; and a parameter file (datafile.dat) includes information specific to the assumed genetic model, such as disease and marker allele frequencies and disease penetrance and dominance relationships. Prior to running any further linkage analysis programs, the UNKNOWN program should be implemented for data checking.

3.1. Example 1: Two-Point Linkage Analysis of an Autosomal-Dominant Disease

In Example 1, we demonstrate two-point linkage analysis using five markers that are linked to a disease locus. Based on the pedigree characteristics (**Fig. 1**), we assume that the disease follows an autosomal-dominant mode of inheritance.

3.1.1. Prepare the Pedigree File

The program MAKEPED translates a "pre-MAKEPED pedigree file" into the LINKAGE format file. The "pre-MAKEPED pedigree file" can be prepared by the user with a text editor, which includes the following columns:
Field 1 = family number
Field 2 = individual number
Field 3 = father number
Field 4 = mother number
Field 5 = sex (1 = male; 2 = female)
Field 6 = affection status (in this case, affected = 2, unaffected = 1, and unknown = 0)

Field 7 = first allele for marker 1
Field 8 = second allele for marker 1

Note: zeros are the default for missing values; every family member takes one record (line); and, although this example involves only one pedigree, multiple pedigrees may be included in the pre-MAKEPED file.

Let the pre-MAKEPED file be marker1.pre. We produce the post-MAKEPED file by typing the Makeped command followed by the names of the input file and the output file: c:\linkage\example1 >makeped marker1.pre marker1.ped. The resulting LINKAGE format pedigree file is as shown in **Textbox 1**.

Family number	Individual number	Father ID	Mother ID	Pointer 1	Pointer 2	Pointer 3	Sex	Proband	Affection status	Allele 1	Allele 2		
1	1	0	0	3	0	0	1	0	0	0	0	Ped: 1	Per: 1
1	2	0	0	3	0	0	2	0	0	0	0	Ped: 1	Per: 2
1	3	1	2	5	9	9	1	0	2	5	8	Ped: 1	Per: 3
1	4	0	0	5	0	0	2	0	1	1	4	Ped: 1	Per: 4
...	...	...	...	...	...	...	...	...	...	...	...	...	...
1	24	19	20	0	0	0	2	0	2	5	5	Ped: 1	Per: 24

Textbox 1. Post-MAKEPED pedigree file for Example 1.

Note: (1) at the program prompt, you will be asked whether there are loops in the pedigree: respond with "n," as this pedigree does not contain loops (*see* the LINKAGE documentation for further details on the handling of pedigrees with loops); (2) respond to the program query regarding proband settings (unless a risk calculation is being performed, the program's automatic selection of the proband is sufficient); (3) the "post-MAKEPED" file has three additional pointer fields: Field 5 = identification number of the first offspring (pointer 1), Field 6 = identification number of the first (or next) paternal sibling (pointer 2), and Field 7 = identification number of the first (or next) maternal sibling (pointer 3).

3.1.2. Prepare the Parameter File

The parameter file can be prepared using either a text editor or the LINK-AGE program PREPLINK. A parameter file for analysis of the pedigree vs marker 1 is shown in **Textbox 2**. Note that:

```
Line1 2 0 0 5  << No. OF LOCI, RISK LOCUS, SEXLINKED (IF 1) PROGRAM
Line2 0 0.0 0.0 0  <<MUT LOCUS, MUT MALE, MUT FEM, HAP FREQ (IF 1)
Line3 1 2  << ORDER OF LOCI
Line4 1 2 << AFFECTION, NO. OF ALLELES
Line5 0.990000 0.010000 << GENE FREQUENCIES
Line6 1  << NO. OF LIABILITY CLASSES
Line7 0.000001 0.999999 0.999999  << PNENETRANCES
Line8 3 8 # mark5 << ALLELE NUMBERS, NO. OF ALLELES
Line9 0.125 0.125 0.125 0.125 0.125 0.125 0.125 0.125 << ALLELE FREQUENCIES
Line10 0 0 << SEX DIFFERENCE, INTERFERENCE (IF 1 OR 2)
Line11 0.0 << RECOMBINATION VALUES
Line12 1 0.01 0.45 << RECOMBINATION VARIED, INCREMENT, FINISHED VALUE
```

Textbox 2. Parameter file for Example 1.

1. Line 1, Field 4: Program codes are 1 for CILINK, 2 for CMAP, 3 for ILINK, 4 for LINKMAP, 5 for MLINK, 6 for LODSCORE, 7 for CLODSCORE. *See* LINK-AGE documentation for a detailed description of each of these programs.
2. Lines 4 to 7 define the trait (disease) locus and lines 8 and 9 describe the marker locus. For this example, the trait locus has two alleles with frequencies as shown. The trait is an autosomal dominant trait with 99.9999% penetrance and pheno-copy rate of 0.000001; consequently, only one liability class has been defined. Marker locus has eight equal-frequent alleles.
3. In reality, allele frequencies for the trait locus (line 5) can be calculated from information obtained either from the literature, or from a source such as the Online Mendelian Inheritance in Man *(6)* (http://www3.ncbi.nlm.nih.gov/omim). Likewise, marker allelic frequencies can be obtained either from the literature or public databases for the population that the pedigree refers to.
4. Line 11 is the genetic distance between the two loci, either assumed or estab-lished.
5. Line 12 specifies variations of the only recombination rate to be tested.

3.1.3. Perform the Analysis

Implementation of the linkage analysis is straightforward. First, copy the pedigree and parameter files into the input files expected by the programs.
>copy marker1.ped pedfile.dat
>copy marker1.dat datafile.dat
Then, invoke the programs in the following order:

>unknown
>mlink

The default output file name is outfile.dat. The screen capture for a marker is shown in **Textbox 3**. For this example, the peaked lod score (3.729, *see* **Table 1**) is obtained at marker 3, which is interpreted to attain the genome-wide significant level.

3.2. Example 2: Multipoint Linkage Analysis by Use of Nearby Markers to Define the Disease Location

In Example 2, we demonstrate the usage of LINKMAP for multipoint link-age analysis of three markers and a disease locus segregating in a hypothetical four-generation pedigree (**Fig. 2**), i.e., identifying the location of the disease gene relative to the markers. This analysis assumes that the genetic map for the markers is spaced with a 10-cM interval, and has been genotyped for all the individuals in the pedigree.

3.2.1. Prepare the Pedigree File

The pedigree file can be prepared in the same way as in Example 1. Now, we deal with the linkage analysis of multiple markers simultaneously. In this pedigree file (either the pre-MAKEPED or post-MAKEPED format), geno-types for each marker are listed on the same line, in the marker order specified in the parameter file.

3.2.2. Prepare the Parameter File

The parameter file can be made either manually or automatically by the linkage control program (LCP) utility included in the LINKAGE package. The parameter file in Example 2 is shown in **Textbox 4**, with a brief description of each line. This example is modified from published data and the marker allelic frequency data are thus used. The same configurations for the disease locus as in Example 1 are used. Note that the multipoint linkage program LINKMAP can be modified and recompiled to suit the problem under consideration (as well as to reduce computational requirements), using the Turbo Pascal com-piler (*see* the LINKAGE documentation and **ref. 7** for details).

3.2.3. Perform the Analysis

To determine the most likely location of the disease gene relative to the marker map, LINKMAP calculates the multipoint likelihoods for some pre-defined locations of the disease locus with the marker map. Usually, one would want to calculate the likelihoods for a set of disease locus positions across the marker map, in each interval. It is painful to have to manually edit the param-

```
Length of real variables =              8 bytes
LINKAGE (V5.1) WITH  2-POINT AUTOSOMAL DATA
 ORDER OF LOCI:   1  2
-----------------------------------
-----------------------------------
THETAS  0.500
-----------------------------------
PEDIGREE |  LN LIKE  | LOG 10 LIKE
-----------------------------------
         1   -54.559539   -23.694907
-----------------------------------
TOTALS       -54.559539   -23.694907
-2 LN(LIKE) =  1.09119078764420794e+02 LOD SCORE =       0.000000
-----------------------------------
-----------------------------------
THETAS  0.000
-----------------------------------
PEDIGREE |  LN LIKE  | LOG 10 LIKE
-----------------------------------
         1   -45.973573   -19.966069
-----------------------------------
TOTALS       -45.973573   -19.966069
-2 LN(LIKE) =  9.19471454422943178e+01 LOD SCORE =       3.728838
-----------------------------------
-----------------------------------
THETAS  0.010
-----------------------------------
PEDIGREE |  LN LIKE  | LOG 10 LIKE
-----------------------------------
         1   -46.121128   -20.030152
-----------------------------------
TOTALS       -46.121128   -20.030152
-2 LN(LIKE) =  9.22422569897523732e+01 LOD SCORE =       3.664755
-----------------------------------

.......................................................................

-----------------------------------
THETAS  0.440
-----------------------------------
PEDIGREE |  LN LIKE  | LOG 10 LIKE
-----------------------------------
         1   -53.625619   -23.289310
-----------------------------------
TOTALS       -53.625619   -23.289310
-2 LN(LIKE) =  1.07251237558302376e+02 LOD SCORE =       0.405597
-----------------------------------
```

Textbox 3. Output of two-point linkage analysis.

Table 1
Results of Two-Point Linkage Profiles in Example 1

Marker	Thetas						
	0.00	0.01	0.05	0.1	0.2	0.3	0.4
Marker1	−3.120	0.842	1.389	1.490	1.350	1.022	0.564
Marker2	3.680	3.617	3.358	3.021	2.303	1.522	0.710
Marker3	3.729	3.665	3.403	3.063	2.336	1.545	0.719
Marker4	1.133	1.777	2.159	2.136	1.762	1.207	0.565
Marker5	0.544	0.527	.0461	0.379	0.222	0.095	0.020

eter file and go through the analysis steps again and again. To start the analysis, type at the DOS prompt:

>linkmap

The output from the analysis is found in a file called "final.out" (as shown in **Textbox 5**). The program does not produce the actual multipoint lod scores directly. One can obtain the multipoint lod scores based on the information in the output file, i.e., by subtracting the log10 likelihood when the disease is linked (with some recombination rates) with the fixed map of markers from the likelihood when the disease is unlinked to the fixed map of markers. Alternatively, LINKLODS will perform the subtraction automatically (*see* LINKAGE documentation for details) and produce a lod score report (**Textbox 6**). The multipoint linkage profile of three markers for this example is depicted in **Fig. 3**.

3.3. Example 3: HOMOG\Heterogeneity Lod Score Computation

In this example, we demonstrate the heterogeneity linkage analysis for an autosomal dominant disease. In addition to the performance of two-point linkage analysis, the example demonstrates the use of the HOMOG computer program. Two families used in this example are shown in **Fig. 4**. The frequency of the disease allele is 0.001, and penetrance is set at 0.95 and phenocopy at 0.005. For demonstration, only one marker is analyzed.

3.3.1. Prepare Pedigree and Parameter Files

The pedigree file for multiple pedigrees can be prepared and formatted in a way similar to that described in Example 1. There are no lines separating the families in the pre-MAKEPED file, and individual numbers can be repeated from pedigree to pedigree, but must be unique within a pedigree. Prior to heterogeneity lod score computation, a two-point linkage analysis for each family must be performed, as HOMOG uses the linkage results as its input file. The two-point linkage analysis can be performed as described in Example 1. Note

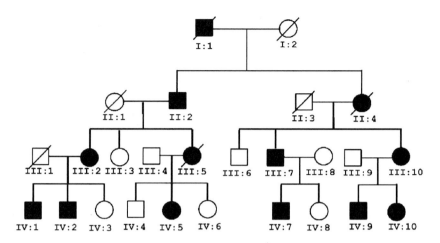

Fig. 2. Pedigree of an artificial family in Example 2.

```
Line1  4 0 0 4 << NO. OF LOCI, RISK LOCUS, SEXLINKED (IF 1) PROGRAM
Line2  0 0.0 0.0 0 << MUT LOCUS, MUT RATE, HAPLOTYPE FREQUENCIES (IF 1)
Line3  1   2 3 4 << ORDER OF LOCI
Line4  1   2   # TRAIT
Line5  0.9900 0.0100 << GENE FREQUENCIES
Line6  1 << NO. OF LIABILITY CLASSES
Line7  0.000 0.800 0.800 << PENETRANCES
Line8  3   4 # marker2
Line9  0.30 0.30 0.05 0.35 << GENE FREQUENCIES
Line10 3   3 # marker3
Line11 0.40 0.10 0.50 << GENE FREQUENCIES
Line12 3   3 # marker4
Line13 0.05 0.40 0.55 << GENE FREQUENCIES
Line14 0 0 << SEX DIFFERENCE, INTERFERENCE (IF 1 OR 2)
Line15 0.50 0.03 0.05 << RECOMBINATION VALUES
Line16 1 0.0 10 << LOCUS VARIED, FINISHING VALUE, NO. OF EVALUATIONS
```

Textbox 4. Parameter file for Example 2.

that MLINK does not provide lod scores for each family separately. LINKLODS can be used to generate family-specific scores.

3.3.2. Perform Homogeneity Testing and Heterogeneity Lod Score Computation

The hypotheses to be considered are:

H1: All families are linked to the marker (linkage homogeneity).

H2: Only some of the families are linked to the marker (linkage heterogeneity).

The likelihood ratio statistic is formulated as follows:

```
THETAS   0.500 0.030 0.050
------------------------------------
PEDIGREE |  LN LIKE  | LOG 10 LIKE
------------------------------------
            1   -101.824193    -44.221685
------------------------------------
TOTALS       -101.824193    -44.221685
-2 LN(LIKE) =   2.03648385478223977e+02
------------------------------------
------------------------------------


.........................................................


THETAS   0.050 0.030 0.050
------------------------------------
PEDIGREE |  LN LIKE  | LOG 10 LIKE
------------------------------------
            1    -92.730405    -40.272303
------------------------------------
TOTALS        -92.730405    -40.272303
-2 LN(LIKE) =   1.85460810500406986e+02
------------------------------------
------------------------------------
THETAS   0.000 0.030 0.050
------------------------------------
PEDIGREE |  LN LIKE  | LOG 10 LIKE
------------------------------------
            1    -91.874728    -39.900688
------------------------------------
TOTALS        -91.874728    -39.900688
-2 LN(LIKE) =   1.83749456560203666e+02
```

Textbox 5. Output of multipoint linkage analysis.

$$\chi^2 = 2\left[\ln L\left(\alpha, \theta_i\right) - \operatorname{Ln} L\left(\alpha = 1.0,\, \theta_0\right)\right]$$

where α is the proportion of linked families, θ_i is the value of the recombination fraction at which the lod score is maximized jointly at θ and α, and θ_0 is the maximum likelihood estimate of θ under linkage homogeneity. This statistic is asymptotically distributed as χ^2 with one degree of freedom.

```
THETAS  0.450  0.030  0.050
Male map position:   -1.1513 (Haldane)   -0.7361 (Kosambi)
      PED         LOD
        1       0.409
   TOTALS       0.409

.......................................................................

THETAS  0.050  0.030  0.050
Male map position:   -0.0527 (Haldane)   -0.0502 (Kosambi)
      PED         LOD
        1       3.949
   TOTALS       3.949

THETAS  0.000  0.030  0.050
Male map position:   -0.0000 (Haldane)   -0.0000 (Kosambi)
      PED         LOD
        1       4.321
   TOTALS       4.321
```

Textbox 6. Lod scores of multipoint linkage analysis.

The input file (say homog.dat) for the HOMOG program for this example is shown in **Textbox 7**. It shows that two-point load scores of 1.70 and 2.02 are obtained at $\theta = 0.01$ for the two families, respectively.

To run the HOMOG program, type:

>homog homog.data homog.out

We explain the output file (as shown in **Textbox 8**) as follows:

❶ A program header that defines the variables α and θ.

❷ The user-specified lod scores and θ values.

❸ A grid of natural log likelihoods calculated from the lod scores provided by the user across various values of α and θ. The first column of this table gives the α values and the last row shows the θ values.

❹ A table of maximum *ln* likelihood values over α given a specified θ value. Note that this value is the highest *ln* likelihood in each column.

❺ A summary of the information described in ❸.

❻ χ^2 tests of significance. Note that the test for linkage heterogeneity (H2 vs H1) shows null ($c^2 = 0$; $p = 1.0$). However, the test for linkage (H1 vs H0) is significant ($\chi^2 = 17.133$; $p = 3.5E\text{-}5$).

❼ The two-unit support interval about the maximum likelihood estimates of α and θ.

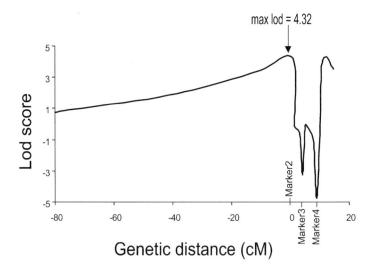

Fig 3. Graph of multipoint lod score from Example 2, with genetic distance in centiMorgens on the *x*-axis, plotted vs the lod score on the *y*-axis. The horizontal line corresponds to lod score of 3.0.

❽ The posterior probabilities that each of the families is "of the linked type" and approximate confidence intervals about these probabilities. For instance, the probabilities that the two families are "of the linked type" is high (100%) and the confidence limits about this estimate are relatively small, indicating that the precision of the estimate is good.

4. Other Linkage Analysis Programs

SAGE 5.0 *(10)* is a package of computer programs for segregation and (model-free and model-based) linkage analysis. The linkage analysis portions of the package are called LODLINK, SIBPAL, LODPAL, and MLOD. SAGE will run under UNIX, Linux, and Windows operating systems. SAGE is freely available for nonprofit organizations, and information can be obtained via the Human Genetic Analysis Resource website at Case Western Reserve University (http://darwin.cwru.edu).

FASTLINK *(11)* is a compilation of the LINKAGE programs that have been improved to speed the calculations, often by as much as an order of magnitude. FASTLINK is available at no charge to the user at http://www.ncbi.nlm.nih.gov/CBBresearch/Schaffer/fastlink.html.

GENEHUNTER *(12)* performs rapid multipoint linkage analysis for parametric lod scores in small pedigrees. Although the pedigree size restriction can

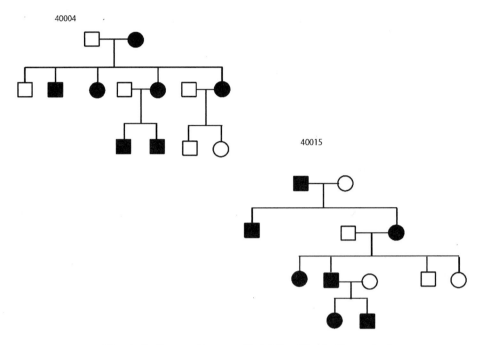

Fig. 4. Pedigree of two artificial families in Example 3.

```
Line1 RLS-40004&40015 << A title line
Line2 5 0.05  95  << No of recombination for lod score computation, step
      size of alpha and the 95% confidence interval to compute
Line3 3 0 80 << An option for output, the smallest alpha and the line length
      of output
Line4 0.01 0.05 0.1 0.2 0.3 << the theta values for lod score
Line5 2 << number of families
Line6 1.695835 1.541498 1.379520 1.031307 0.655244 <<lod scores for family 1
Line7 2.024560 1.857002 1.683365 1.316463 0.919947 <<lod scores for family 2
```

Textbox 7. Parameter file for Example 3.

be cumbersome, GENEHUNTER allows many markers to be run simulta-neously, thereby allowing for whole-chromosome multipoint analyses.

SimWalk2 *(13)*, now in version 2.91, is a statistical genetics computer application for haplotype, parametric linkage, nonparametric linkage (NPL), identity by descent (IBD), and mistyping analyses on any size of pedigree. SimWalk2 uses Markov chain Monte Carlo (MCMC) and simulated annealing algorithms to perform these multipoint analyses. Parametric linkage analysis is

```
Program  HOMOG  version 3.35   J. Ott❶
Heterogeneity: two family types, one with linkage, one without
  alpha  = proportion of families with linkage (theta<1/2)
  1-alpha= proportion of families without linkage (theta=1/2)

>> RLS-40004&40015 <<

  Fam.  Lod scores❷
     1   1.70   1.54   1.38   1.03   0.66
     2   2.02   1.86   1.68   1.32   0.92
  Theta  0.01   0.05   0.10   0.20   0.30

  Alpha ln L(alpha,theta) ❸
  1.00   8.57   7.83   7.05   5.41   3.63
  0.95   8.47   7.72   6.95   5.31   3.54
  0.90   8.36   7.62   6.85   5.21   3.45
.....................................................................
  0.15   4.93   4.26   3.58   2.28   1.16
  0.10   4.21   3.57   2.94   1.77   0.85
  0.05   3.06   2.50   1.98   1.08   0.47
  Theta  0.01   0.05   0.10   0.20   0.30

Table of conditional max. Ln(L) over alpha's, given theta or x❹
     theta or x alpha max   Max.Ln(L)  Lik. ratio
  1    0.0100    1.0000    8.5665 5252.8501
  2    0.0500    1.0000    7.8253 2503.2257
  3    0.1000    1.0000    7.0526 1155.8062
  4    0.2000    1.0000    5.4059  222.7255
  5    0.3000    1.0000    3.6270   37.6003

                                       Estimates of❺
Hypotheses                        Max.lnL    Alpha    Theta
H2: Linkage, heterogeneity         8.5665   1.0000   0.0100
H1: Linkage, homogeneity           8.5665     (1)    0.0100
H0: No linkage                       (0)      (0)     (99)

Components of chi-square❻
Source                             df  Chi-square    L ratio
H2 vs. H1  Heterogeneity            1       0.000     1.0000
H1 vs. H0  Linkage                  1      17.133  5252.8501
H2 vs. H0  Total                    2      17.133  5252.8501

 2.00-unit support intervals (LR =    7.3891):❼
Alpha     0.4000     1.0000
Theta     0.0100     0.1000

Family   Conditional prob.       Support limits❽
  no.     of linked type       lower      upper
   1            1.0000         0.9707     1.0000
   2            1.0000         0.9860     1.0000
```

Textbox 8. Results from HOMOG analysis of data in Example 3.

performed in order to obtain location scores, i.e., the likelihood of several putative positions among the marker loci for the trait locus. These location scores are directly comparable with multipoint lod scores and are presented in log10 units.

MEGA2 (http://watson.hgen.pitt.edu/docs/mega2_html/mega2.html) is not a linkage analysis but is used in data management. It allows for facile manipulation of genetic data into parameter files appropriate for use in a variety of linkage analysis software packages.

Acknowledgments

This work was supported by National Institutes of Health (NIH) grants R01 HL65630, R01 HL66251, P50 HL77107, and an American Heart Association Established Investigator award (to Q. K. W.).

Further Reading

1. Ott's *Analysis of Human Genetic Linkage (8)* is a necessary reference book for human genetic linkage analysis, with both theoretical and practical perspectives.
2. Terwilliger and Ott's *Handbook of Human Genetic Linkage (7)* is a nice hands-on guidebook for performing human linkage analysis.
3. Speer, in "Use of LINKAGE Programs for Linkage Analysis" *(9)*, presents detailed guidelines for, and seven examples of, model-based linkage analysis, including sex-linked linkage analysis.

References

1. Griffiths, A. J. F., Miller, J. H., Suzuki, D. T., Lewontin, R. C., and Gelbart, W. M. (1993) *An Introduction to Genetic Analysis*, W. H. Freeman and Company, New York.
2. Morton, N. E. (1955) Sequential tests for the detection of linkage. *Am. J. Hum. Genet.* **7**, 277–318.
3. Conneally, P. M., Edwards, J. H., Kidd, K. K., et al. (1985) Report of the Committee on Methods of Linkage Analysis and Reporting. *Cytogenet. Cell Genet.* **40**, 356–359.
4. Ott, J., Bhattacharya, S., Chen, J. D., et al. (1990) Localizing multiple X chromosome-linked retinitis pigmentosa loci using multilocus homogeneity tests. *Proc. Natl. Acad. Sci. USA* **87**, 701–704.
5. Bhat, A., Heath, S. C., and Ott, J. (1999) Heterogeneity for multiple disease loci in linkage analysis. *Hum. Hered.* **49**, 229–231.
6. McKusick, V. (1992) *Mendelian Inheritance in Man,* Johns Hopkins University Press, Baltimore, MD.
7. Terwilliger, J. D. and Ott, J. (1994) *Handbook of Human Genetic Linkage*, Johns Hopkins University Press, Baltimore, MD.

8. Ott, J. (1999) *Analysis of Human Genetic Linkage,* Johns Hopkins University Press, Baltimore, MD.

9. Speer, M. C. (1995) Use of LINKAGE Programs for Linkage Analysis, in *Current Protocols in Human Genetics,* (Dracopoli, N. C., Haines, J. L., Korf, B. R., et al., eds.), John Wiley and Sons, New York, NY, pp. 1.7.1–1.7.53.

10. Statistical Analysis for Genetic Epidemiology (S.A.G.E.) 5.0. (2004) Available from the Department of Epidemiology and Biostatistics, Case Western Reserve University, Cleveland, OH.

11. Cottingham, R. W., Jr., Idury, R. M., and Schaffer, A. A. (1993) Faster sequential genetic linkage computations. *Am. J. Hum. Genet.* **53,** 252–263.

12. Kruglyak, L., Daly, M. J., Reeve-Daly, M. P., and Lander, E. S. (1996) Parametric and nonparametric linkage analysis: a unified multipoint approach. *Am. J. Hum. Genet.* **58,** 1347–1363.

13. Sobel, E. and Lange, K. (1996) Descent graphs in pedigree analysis: applications to haplotyping, location scores, and marker-sharing statistics. *Am. J. Hum. Genet.* **58,** 1323–1337.

6

SAGE Programs

Model-Free Linkage Analysis for Complex Cardiovascular Phenotypes

Shaoqi Rao and Qing K. Wang

Summary

A complex disease trait refers to a phenotype that does not follow simple Mendelian segregation attributable to a single gene locus, but instead may be caused by multiple disease loci, their interactions, polygenic inheritance, and environmental effects. Most cardiovascular disorders are thought to have a polygenic basis with complex interactions with environmental factors. A gene that increases or decreases the risk to a complex cardiovascular disease (susceptibility gene) can now be mapped to a specific chromosomal region by model-free linkage analysis, and follow-up molecular genetic studies can identify the specific gene at the locus. This chapter describes a protocol for model-free linkage analysis of a complex trait, as implemented in the popular genetic analysis software—SAGE. In particular, the Haseman-Elston sib-pair regression method is introduced and implemented with examples to demonstrate how to identify susceptibility loci for complex traits.

Key Words: Complex traits; model-free linkage analysis; Haseman-Elston regression; identity-by-descent; cardiovascular disease.

1. Genetic Concepts and Background

We start this chapter by introducing the relevant genetic concepts and background for understanding and implementing a model-free linkage analysis. Examples illustrating the application of the Statistical Analysis for Genetic Epidemiology (SAGE) programs (PEDINFO, FREQ, MARKERINFO, RELTEST, GENIBD, and SIBPAL) are then provided to elucidate the step-by-step protocol for performing Haseman-Elston (H-E) sib-pair regression. It should be noted that the majority of forms of cardiovascular disorders are quantitative traits, although they are phenotypically binary or ordinal. Methods for

From: *Methods in Molecular Medicine, Vol. 128: Cardiovascular Disease; Methods and Protocols; Volume 1*
Edited by: Q. Wang © Humana Press Inc., Totowa, NJ

studying continuously distributed cardiovascular phenotypes (e.g., lipid profiles) are not different from what are described here as examples of a binary phenotype. In other words, the procedures outlined for the H-E regression can be applied to either quantitative or qualitative data. We conclude this chapter with suggestions for further reading and alternative approaches.

1.1. Complex Traits

We use the term "complex trait" to refer to a biological phenotype with an unknown mode of inheritance. The same confounding factors that influence monogenic linkage analysis also complicate the genetic mapping of complex traits, for example, genetic heterogeneity, phenotypic misclassification, penetrance, and so on. It is generally believed that complex traits have moderate to high environmental influence, plus polygenic backgrounds that blur the Mendelian dominant or recessive inheritance of a major gene segregating in the pedigrees. It can also be the case that a subset of families could be owing to a single Mendelian locus, whereas others are due to different loci. In short, a simple correspondence between the genotype (genetic endowment) and phenotype (observable manifestation) breaks down, which can arise from a list of factors: (1) incomplete penetrance, including variable age of onset; (2) difficulties in phenotypic definition; (3) phenocopy; (4) genetic heterogeneity; (5) polygenic inheritance; (6) high frequency of disease-causing alleles; and (7) other genetic mechanisms. The genes involved in a complex trait (also called a polygenic or multifactorial trait) are often referred to as "susceptibility genes" because they can significantly increase or decrease a risk for the individuals who carry the genes. This is in distinction to the term "causative genes," used in genetic studies of monogenic disorders, which refers to genes that lead directly to the clinical disease phenotype when mutated.

1.2. Genetic Model-Based vs Model-Free Linkage Analysis

The methods of genetic analysis for a complex trait are different from the strategies for monogenic Mendelian disorder (e.g., as described in the LINKAGE package). All of the approaches to linkage analysis can be divided into two types: model-based and model-free. The model-based approach requires an assumption of a genetic model as well as specification of certain parameters (e.g., mode of inheritance of a trait, allelic models (number and frequencies) of the trait and the markers, mutation rate, and penetrance *(1)*. Model-based linkage analysis method is the most powerful method for identification of a disease locus/gene, provided that the underlying genetic model and other parameters are specified correctly. Statistical power is decreased, often severely, when the wrong assumptions about the genetic model are made.

In contrast, genetic model-free linkage analysis does not require prior knowledge of the parameters that define the genetic model for a complex disease. However, it does require accurate definition of the disease phenotype and evidence of genetic contributions to its underlying pathogenesis. The determination of the genetic component of a complex human disease will perhaps continue to be a critical issue, as human pedigrees are often ascertained from the clinical settings and the sampling schemes may not be defined by any single ascertainment form. Nevertheless, genetic analysis of the collected samples for evidence of genetic factors, as a requisite step toward identification of disease genes by model-free linkage analysis, cannot be ignored. Without familial aggregation, in which genetic factors play an important role, the expense and effort involved in further gene mapping and cloning would be wasted *(2,3)*. A variety of methods and approaches have been developed for exploring the genetic basis of a complex disease, including family history, familial aggregation, complex segregation analysis, and variance component analysis of pedigree data. The SAGE program FCOR is specifically designed to perform this kind of genetic analysis by estimating familial correlations between various familial relation types. This chapter describes the protocol for linkage analysis of a complex disease by assuming either that genetic evidence for the complex disease has been well documented or that one has performed a data analysis of the pedigree samples and identified strong evidence of genetic involvement in the recruited samples. Among the number of model-free linkage approaches available, the identical-by-descent (IBD) allele-sharing-based method is the most popular for exploring the relations between the genetic sharing and phenotypic sharing between the familial relatives (e.g., sib pairs). In the sib-pair method described in this chapter, IBD relationships are used in examining allele sharing among siblings. Extensions and derivatives using other familial relations or restriction of the analysis to only affected individuals have been seen in the literature. Although genetic model-free methods are less powerful in their ability to detect linkage than model-based methods (under optimal conditions), genetic model-free methods are the only comprehensive and unbiased approach, especially when the underlying genetic model is unknown.

1.3. Identity-by-State and Identity-by-Descent

All methods that have been developed for mapping complex traits in human sib pairs or other relations depend on the concepts of identity-by-state (IBS) and IBD. IBS describes the state in which a pair of individuals shares the same variant of some allelic systems. In other words, two alleles are IBS if they cannot be distinguished by means of a particular method of detection. IBD, on the other hand, requires not only that the alleles appear the same on a gel or by another polymorphism detection method, but also that the allele(s) for a relative pair are derived or inherited from a common ancestor. Clearly, IBD is a subset of the concept of IBS, i.e., alleles of IBS are not necessarily IBD, but alleles that are shared IBD must also be IBS. Determination of IBS for the alleles between a relative pair is straightforward, whereas IBD computation can be much complicated for complex and multigeneration pedigrees and when multiple loci are considered simultaneously. The SAGE GENGIBD program is specifically designed to perform the analysis.

If a locus is located on some autosome and follows a Mendelian inheritance pattern (i.e., without segregation distortion), an average of one-fourth of sib pairs will share two alleles IBD, half will share one allele IBD, and one-fourth will share no alleles IBD. These values are also expected for a sib pair if considering the average proportion of autosomal genetic material as a whole, which is also defined to be the kinship coefficient in the traditional quantitative genetics. In variance-component linkage analysis of complex diseases, the kinship coefficients for different relative types are used to model the residual genetic covariance functions. In the context of model-free linkage analysis, we often mean the term IBD by results obtained from analysis of a specific genomic region (e.g., a marker or group of markers). In essence, linkage evidence is identified by a significant departure of the IBD value(s) at some genomic region from the expected value (the genomic average) for a relative pair.

IBD is often presented as the estimated proportion of alleles $\hat{\pi}$ shared by a specific relative type (e.g., sib pair). This estimate is derived by calculating the sum of the probability that the pair shares two alleles IBD plus 0.5 times the probability that the pair shares one allele IBD. **Figure 1** shows an example for computation of IBD between members of a sib pair using an artificial nuclear family with mating type of AB × CD. In this particular case (all four alleles of parents are distinct), IBS estimate for the sib pair is the same as IBD, as the origins of the alleles in the sib pair can be determined unambiguously.

1.4. H-E Sib-Pair Regression

The H-E method was originally developed for quantitative traits *(4)*, but has been adapted for use with qualitative traits. Suppose that χ_{ij} is the phenotype (either continuous or discrete value) for the *j*th sibling ($j = 1,2$) in the *i*th pair from a pedigree. In the original formulation of H-E, the test uses the squared sib-pair trait difference, $y_i = (\chi_{i1} - \chi_{i2})^2$, as the transformed phenotype to capture the phenotypic similarity (or difference) of the relative pair. Then, the values of y_i are regressed on a marker $\hat{\pi}$, where *i* indexes the sib pair to reveal the relationship between genetic and phenotypic similarity for the familial siblings. Both intercept (α) and the regression coefficient (β) are a function of the

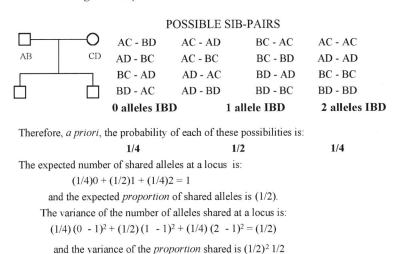

Fig. 1. Sample pedigree for illustrating identity-by-descent computation of a sib pair.

recombination fraction (between the putative genetic locus and observed marker) and the genetic variance attributable to the genetic locus that is linked to the marker being considered *(5)*:

$$\text{Expectation}(\alpha) = \sigma_e^2 + 2\left[\theta^2 + \left(1 - \theta^2\right)\right]\sigma_g^2, \text{ and Expection}(\beta) = -2\left(1 - 2\theta\right)^2 \sigma_g^2$$

where σ_e^2 and σ_g^2 are the respective environmental and genetic variances of the trait under study, and θ is the recombination fraction. A significantly negative estimate of β indicates linkage between the marker locus and the trait locus that influences the trait, and the corresponding point-wise *p* value can be obtained using an asymptotic *t*-test. The basic idea underlying the method is that sib pairs that are identical by descent at a marker locus will be phenotypically similar for the traits influenced by a nearby linked gene.

Recent time has witnessed increasing attempts to improve the statistical power for the original H-E regression test. In 1997, Wright *(6)* showed that the original phenotypic formulation (squared trait difference) ignores the information available in the sib-pair trait sum. Maximum likelihood using a multivariate normal distribution to model the individual sibling values, rather than just the pair differences, leads to appreciably more power *(7,8)* in the case of a continuous trait. In 1995, Single and Finch *(9)* showed that when sibships of size larger than two are analyzed, increased power is obtained when a generalized least-squares regression is performed to allow for the correlations between the pairs of squared sib-pair trait differences. Therefore, in the modified H-E regression, the SAGE developers have extended the original sib-pair regression to allow for both covariates and multiple loci and their interactions in a computationally fast manner. The new H-E regression also capitalizes on the fact that the squared mean corrected sib-pair sum is also linearly related in a very similar manner to the proportion of marker alleles shared IBD. In detail, the new H-E regression program SIBPAL has incorporated the following extension:

1. The model is extended to a more involved form of a general linear model:

$$y = \alpha + \sum_i a_i \hat{\pi}_i + \sum_j d_j \hat{f}_{2j} + \sum_k c_k f(z_k) + \varepsilon ,$$

where α is the intercept, d_j is the dominant genetic variance owing to the jth marker, a_i is the additive genetic variance due to the ith marker, c_k is a nuisance parameter accounting for the effect of some function f of the kth covariate, and ε is the residual error.

2. Several extended dependent variables (the quadratic forms of the siblings' phenotypes) have been used. Let the sib-pair trait values be χ_{1j} and χ_{2j} for the jth sib pair used ($j = 1, 2, ..., n$). For continuous traits, χ_{ij} is simply the value of the trait. For binary traits, $x_{ij} = 1$ if the individual is affected and $x_{ij} = 0$ if the individual is not affected. Then, the dependent variables are:

Trait Difference: $y_{dj} = -\dfrac{1}{2}\left[\left(x_{1j} - \bar{x}\right) - \left(x_{2j} - \bar{x}\right)\right]^2 = -\dfrac{1}{2}\left(x_{1j} - x_{2j}\right)^2$

Trait Sum: $y_{sj} = \dfrac{1}{2}\left[\left(x_{1j} - \bar{x}\right) + \left(x_{2j} - \bar{x}\right)\right]^2$

Trait Product: $y_{pj} = \dfrac{1}{2}\left(y_{dj} + y_{sj}\right) = \left(x_{1j} - \bar{x}\right) \times \left(x_{2j} - \bar{x}\right)$

Trait Weighted: $y_{cj} = \dfrac{1}{2} \dfrac{\text{Var}\left(y_{dj}\right) y_{sj} + \text{Var}\left(y_{sj}\right) y_{dj}}{\text{Var}\left(y_{dj}\right) + \text{Var}\left(y_{sj}\right)}$

Assuming randomly sampled sibships, and a model with a single marker locus linked to the trait locus with recombination fraction θ, the expected value of the dependent variables is:

$$\text{Expectation}(y) = \alpha + (1 - 2\theta)^2 \sigma_g^2 ,$$

or

$$\text{Expectation}(y) = \alpha + (1 - 2\theta)^2 \sigma_a^2 + (1 - 2\theta)^4 \sigma_d^2 .$$

Note that in the newly released SAGE 5.0, further definitions of dependent variables are allowed, including a weighted combination of the dependent variables above. A statistical test of linkage (*t*-test) compares the regression parameters (β = a or d or both) with 0, its value under the null hypothesis of no linkage.

3. In order to account for the polygenic (and common environmental) residuals in the H-E model, the modified model permits a correlated residual matrix. In general, if there are s siblings in a sibship, there are $s(s - 1)/2$ sib pairs and $s^2(s - 1)^2/4$ entries in the correlation matrix for that sibship, of which

$s(s - 1)/2$ are 1 (down the main diagonal);

$s(s - 1)(s - 2)$ are ρ_1 (when one sibling is in common);

$s(s - 1)(s - 2)(s - 3)/4$ are ρ_0 (no siblings in common).

ρ_1 and ρ_0 are correlations that differ depending on the dependent variable.

2. SAGE Programs

The goal of this chapter is to instruct the readers on a general protocol for sib-pair regression analysis for mapping complex diseases, as implemented in the popular software package SAGE. For the full list of programs contained in the software package, the user can consult the SAGE documentation. The most updated version, SAGE 5.0, can be obtained following the instructions on its home page (http://darwin.cwru.edu/sage/index.php), and a member of a non-profit organization can acquire a free license for it.

A flow chart for linkage analysis of a complex trait is depicted in **Fig. 2**, which constitutes a strategic protocol for running the relevant programs available in SAGE. The first step in undertaking a genetic study of a complex trait is to establish evidence for genetic influence, e.g., by familial aggregation analysis using the SAGE program FCOR. It is critical that the genetic basis of the trait is elucidated before the expensive and time-consuming process of data collection and genotyping is begun. Segregation analysis using the SAGE program SEGREG can further characterize the underlying genetic architecture and provide important genetic parameters for linkage analysis, especially for model-based linkage analysis. However, because of the scope of this chapter, we will not illustrate these analyses; rather, we will assume that either that these analyses have been performed or that strong evidence for genetic contribution in the trait under study has been established.

Data quality control and correction of data errors could also be a major undertaking for a large-scale linkage analysis. Essential data cleanings to remove "illegal" data entry (e.g., character data for an item of a numerical nature) or any data entry of "biological error" (outside biological limits) should be performed in ways similar to any large-scale data analysis. However, prior to genetic linkage analysis, additional data cleaning and corrections should be performed (1) to correct any familial relationship errors using the SAGE pro-

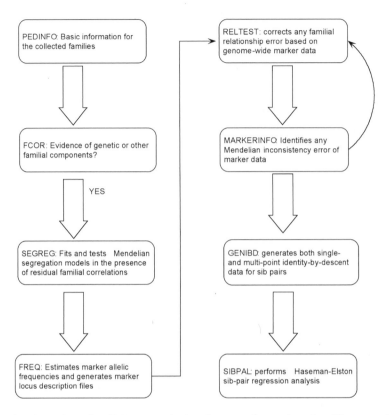

Fig. 2. Flow chart for linkage analysis of a complex trait using Haseman-Elston regression.

gram RELTEST and (2) to correct any errors of Mendelian inconsistencies of marker data using the SAGE program MARKERINFO. It should be noted that there is no optimal sequence for the two data corrections, as they are mutually dependent.

2.1. PEDINFO

PEDINFO (PEDigree INFOrmation) provides many useful descriptive statistics on pedigree data, including means, variances, and histograms of family, sibship, and pedigree size, and counts of each type of relative pairs.

2.2. FCOR

FCOR (Familial CORrelations) calculates multivariate familial correlations with their asymptotic standard errors. This program can calculate both interclass (e.g., parents–offspring) and intraclass (e.g., siblings) for all types of relation pairs available in the pedigrees without assuming multivariate normality of the traits across family members. Technically, this type of analysis is a more detailed version of the mixed linear model approach in that each type of relative pair is estimated separately as opposed to being modeled as a function of a few parameters in a single covariance matrix. Historically, family aggregation analysis has been the most popular method for determining genetic components in a disease manifestation. This method, in essence, is to estimate the correlations between various biological relatives and then similarly assume that they can be parsimoniously explained by an additive genetic contribution and a common household contribution, but without making all of the other assumptions of the mixed linear model.

2.3. SEGREG

SEGREG (SEGREGation models) fits and tests Mendelian segregation models in the presence of residual familial correlations. The trait analyzed can be continuous, binary, or a binary disease trait with variable age of onset. This program can also be used for commingling analysis, to predict the major genotype of any pedigree member, and to prepare penetrance files for model-based linkage analysis.

Regressive multivariate logistic models for binary traits (e.g., most cardiovascular clinical phenotypes) are the most commonly used formulations in the investigation of the segregation pattern within the pedigrees *(10)*, and are based on the regressive model assumption that, as a condition of the phenotype and major type of any individual who belongs to two nuclear families, the likelihoods for those two nuclear families are independent *(11)*. In this model, the marginal probability (called susceptibility) that any pedigree member has a particular phenotype is the same for all members who have the same values of any covariates in the model and is given by the cumulative logistic function:

$$\gamma = \frac{e^{\theta_i w_i}}{1 + e^{\theta_i}},$$

where w_i is the trait value for the ith individual, 1 is the trait value for an affected individual, and 0 is the trait value for an unaffected individual; and θ_i, the logit of the susceptibility for the ith individual, can depend on the major type (u = AA or AB or BB) and covariates $z_{i1}, z_{i2}, ..., z_{iK}$:

$$\theta_u(i) = \beta_u + \zeta_1 z_{i1} + ... + \zeta_k z_{iK}.$$

Nuclear familial residual association parameter (ρ), analogous to the correlation parameter in regressive models for continuous traits *(12)*, is a second-order correlation and is incorporated into the models to account for residual polygenic and common environment effects. Often, no spouse correlation and equal parent–offspring and sib–sib correlation are assumed, but can be varied in the parameter settings for SEGREG. Several methods for ascertainment bias are dependent on the specific sampling scheme(s) from which the pedigrees are recruited.

The program can be used to test the several criteria for inferring a major gene *(13)*: (1) rejection of the hypothesis of no major effects; (2) rejection of the hypothesis of no transmission of major effects; (3) failure to reject the hypothesis of Mendelian transmission; and (4) rejection of hypothesis of any particular Mendelian inheritance models (dominant, recessive, and general Mendelian models) and so on. Hypotheses are assessed by the likelihood ratio test, under the assumption that the negative of twice the difference in natural logarithms for hierarchical models follows a χ^2 distribution *(14)*. The SAGE. program SEGREG estimates following parameters: qA, the frequency of the putative disease allele (A); τ_{AA}, τ_{AB}, τ_{BB} = the probability that an individual of type AA, AB, or BB transmits the A allele to an offspring (for the Mendelian case, these correspond to 1.0, 0.5, and 0.0, respectively); $Susc_{AA}$, $Susc_{AB}$, $Susc_{BB}$ = susceptibility on the logit scale that major type AA, AB, or BB confers a specific risk that an individual with such type develops a clinic binary disease; and the first-degree second-moment familial correlation coefficient (ρ) measuring residual multifactorial (polygenic and common environment) effects.

2.4. FREQ

FREQ (allele FREQuency estimator) estimates allele frequencies from marker data on related individuals with known structure and generates marker locus description files, needed by GENIBD, and other SAGE programs.

2.5. RELTEST

RELationship TESTing employs a Markov process model of allele sharing along the chromosome and classifies pairs of pedigree members according to their true relationship using genome scan data *(15)*. This program currently analyzes four different types of putative pairs: full sib pairs, half sib pairs, parent–offspring pairs, and unrelated marital pairs.

2.6. MAKERINFO

MARKER INFOrmation detects Mendelian inconsistencies of markers in pedigree data.

2.7. GENIBD

GENerate IBD sharing probabilities generates both single- and multipoint IBD distributions using a variety of algorithms tailored for different types of relative pairs in pedigrees. Exact methods can be used for small pedigrees with loops. IBD sharing can also be interpolated between markers.

2.8. SIBPAL

SIBling Pair AnaLysis performs mean tests, proportion tests, and linear regression-based modeling of squared sib-pair differences and mean-corrected sums of a trait as a function of marker allele IBD sharing. Available analyses can use either single- or multipoint IBD information, and models allow for both binary and continuous traits due to multiple genetic loci, including epistatic interactions and covariate effects.

3. Procedures for Linkage Analysis of Complex Traits

In this section, we demonstrate a strategic approach for performing H-E sib-pair regression using the GeneQuest pedigrees collected through the Department of Cardiovascular Medicine at the Cleveland Clinic Foundation *(16,17)*. GeneQuest population consists of 1613 individuals in more than 400 multiplex families with familial premature acute myocardial infarction. Prior to genetic mapping of the complex disease, we performed quantitative genetic analysis to estimate the genetic contribution in the trait using both mixed linear model and familial aggregation analysis, implemented using the SAGE program FCOR. In this ascertained sample, the estimated heritability for the trait, or ratio of the additive genetic variance to the total phenotypic variance, was from 0.27 (estimated using mixed linear model) to 0.65 (based on weighted sibling correlations estimated by FCOR) (Rao, S. and Wang, Q. K., unpublished data). Therefore, in the real example, we will focus on the protocol for the remaining steps illustrated in **Fig. 2**. These recruited pedigrees were genotyped at the National Heart, Lung, and Blood Institute Mammalian Genotyping Facility for 408 markers that span the entire human genome at every 10 cM. For this demonstration, we select the genotype data of seven markers on chromosome 2.

In the PC version of SAGE 5.0, SAGE programs are executed from the provided graphical user interface (GUI), as demonstrated in **Fig. 3**. This GUI provides easy and efficient ways for a user to perform complicated genetic analysis. The left vertical bar (called Components window) lists the current variety of modules included in this package. The top bar provides several menus for managing, viewing, and analyzing data files. Two other "view" windows (Tasks and Consol, as captured) can be used to monitor the process of the runs. All the analysis starts with definition of a project and separate analysis is

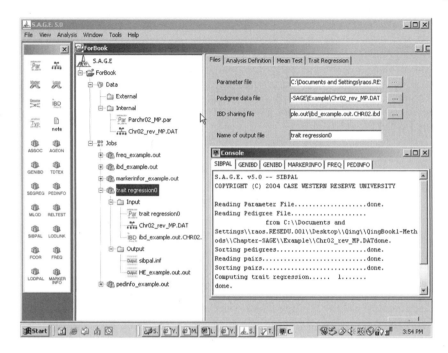

Fig. 3. Graphical user interface (GUI) for the Statistical Analysis for Genetic Epidemiology (SAGE) 5.0 program.

performed as a job (the five jobs for this example are shown in **Fig. 3**). A user can resort to the GUI to prepare the needed data files or made manually. The settings for different analyses can be figured out in the parameter file or interactively made by using the GUI.

3.1. Data Preparation

Each SAGE program requires several input files in order to run. The following is a list of the input files that are required to run one or other programs used in this example: (1) parameter file, (2) pedigree data file, (3) marker locus description file, (4) genome description file, and (5) IBD sharing file.

3.1.1. Parameter File

The parameter file contains a list of instructions that a user defines as his/her own options for performing a genetic analysis using SAGE programs. Then, SAGE reads these instructions to determine (1) how to interpret the contents of the given pedigree data file, (2) how many different analyses have been requested, and (3) which options have been specified for each analysis.

A parameter file is simply a text file containing a list of SAGE program instructions written according to a specific syntax. It should be noted that a single parameter file may be used to specify options for multiple SAGE programs. The parameter file (**Textbox 1**) for this example contains our supplied specifications for five programs. Essentially, the parameter file has two major distinct parts: the data part and the programs part. The list of instructions, also called statements, have the general syntax:

$$\text{parameter}\left[\text{=value}\right]\left[,\text{attribute}\left[=\textbf{value}\right]\right]*\left[\{\left[\textit{statement}\right]*\}\right]$$

in which the square brackets ([]) indicate grouping of optional terms and are not to be entered by the user. The asterisk (*) indicates that the proceeding group or item may be repeated zero or more times. The terms "**parameter**" and "**attribute**" represent SAGE reserved *keywords*, and the braces ({ }) are used to enclose an optional *block* of zero or more statements. For detailed descriptions of the syntax, users can consult with the SAGE documentation or the supporting professionals.

Now, we illustrate the example parameter file:

L1: the title for this run. Note that the insertion of a pound sign (#) here (or at any point of a line) in the parameter file causes SAGE to ignore the remainder of the line, thus helping a user to add *comments* on the contents of a parameter file.

L2: to start pedigree block. SAGE accepts two major data formats: character-delimited or column-delimited. Here we chose the latter.

L3: this statement (FORTRAN Format) instructs how to read the corresponding column-aligned data file, prepared by some data management software (e.g., SAS).

L4: this statement specifies the code for missing pedigree members.

L5: it can also be coded as "M" or "F," respectively.

L6–L10: these five fields are reserved and also necessary for the programs to interpret the familial relationships of the individuals contained in the data. Note that each individual should have a record containing the five fields, even if the parents for the subject are unknown (i.e., code of zero) or the subject does not have any other phenotypic and genotypic data.

L11,L12: SAGE allows inclusion of (multiple) covariates in several models, e.g., the H-E regression models.

L13: SAGE can handle both discrete (in this example) or continuous traits.

L14,L15: SAGE accepts two genotype formats (two alleles are put together or separately). It is cautioned that zeros are not considered to be a missing value in some programs (e.g., FREQ), and thus are not the recommended coding values.

L16: the 14 lines describe the marker data of seven loci. The syntax is slightly different for the two genotype formats; see SAGE documentation for detail.

L17: from this line on are several blocks for five SAGE programs, which will be described later.

```
L1  #Pedigree:CAD: Chr2
    #Column Delimited Pedigree Reader
    #The format is designed to be used by all programs
L2  pedigree, column
    {
    #Specify the format of how various fields are to be read

L3  format="(4(1x,a7),2(1x,a2),1x,a3,1x,a2/14(a4))"

    #field encoding parameters
L4  individual_missing_value="0"
L5  sex_code, male="1", female="2"

    #Family structure, This maps the fields to the data contained in them

L6  pedigree_id
L7  individual_id
L8  parent_id
L9  parent_id
L10 sex_field

    # Traits and covariates
    #covariates
L11 covariate=race, missing="."
L12 covariate=gender, missing="."
    # trait
L13 trait="MI",binary,affected="1",unaffected="2",missing="."

# marker data
L14 #Missing="./."
L15 Missing="."
L16 allele=GATA69E12, missing="."   #First allele of m1
    allele=GATA69E12, missing="."   #Second allele of m1
    allele=GATA88G05, missing="."
    allele=GATA88G05, missing="."
    allele=GATA176C01, missing="."
    allele=GATA176C01, missing="."
    allele=GATA4E11, missing="."
    allele=GATA4E11, missing="."
    allele=GATA27A12, missing="."
    allele=GATA27A12, missing="."
    allele=GATA4D07, missing="."
    allele=GATA4D07, missing="."
    allele=GGAA20G04, missing="."
    allele=GGAA20G04, missing="."
}

L17 pedinfo, out=pedinfo_example.out
{
#each_pedigree=true
#suppress_general=true
}

markerinfo, out=markerinfor_example.out
```

(Textbox 1 continued on next page)

3.1.2. Data File

SAGE data file(s) should exactly correspond to the format specified in the pedigree block in the parameter file regardless of which data format is used. It is critical to assure that the data file(s) has been read and interpreted by SAGE

```
{
#sample_id="the name of a field in the pedigree file"
#consistent_out="true or false for outputting inconsistency symbol []"
}

freq, out=freq_example.out
{
#skip_mle=true #Specify whether to skip ML computation of allele frequencies
}

GENIBD, out=ibd_example.out
{
title="SP" # specify title of the run
ibd_mode="singlepoint" # either singlepoint or multipoint
region=chr02 # the region in genomic description file to be run
#scan_type=intervals #default value is "markers"
#distance=2.0
use_simulation=false # allow simulation on large pedigrees
#split_pedigrees=yes # option to split large pedigrees
}

trait_regression, out=HE_example.out
{
#regression_method=w2 # one of six types of dependent variable
trait=MI # the trait used as the dependent variable
covariate=race # covariate 1
covariate=gender # covariate 2
#compute_empirical_pvalues=true,threshold ="0.00074",max_replicates=100000
#subset="the indicator for using only subset of the data"
}
```

Textbox 1. The parameter file for the example in this chapter.

programs correctly before any analysis is performed. Special attention is given to the coding for missing values and blank fields. In the character-delimited format, it is required that every field has a value (either a real value or a missing value). SAGE programs recognize the character-delimited format(s) via the specific delimiter(s) and the header in the data file that lists all of variables for each record.

The data file (part shown in **Textbox 2**) for this example is prepared according to column format using the SAS software. SAGE recognizes each pedigree variable by its column locations in the data file, as instructed by the FORTRAN format statement in the parameter file (*also see* **Textbox 1**). Hence, a blank field(s) is allowed but not recommended for column-delimited SAGE data files. As shown in **Textbox 2**, each record for each subject in the pedigreed population can occupy multiple lines. In this example, the first line records the basic information (the first five fields) for connecting familial relationships, two covariates and the trait, and the second line the genotypes for seven markers.

Notes: SAGE 5.0 provides a new utility for further processing data file, called a user-defined *function* block, to allow a user to define new trait, phenotype, or covariate variables that are a function(s) of existing pedigree vari-

```
25001    25001    99034    99035   1  3    1  1
3    4   12  12    .    .    3    6   2    5    5   10    6    7
25001    25002    99034    99035   2  3    2  2
3    3   12  13    .    .    4    6   3    4    5   10    6    7
25001    25170    99034    99035   1  3    1  .
4    5   12  13    4    6    3   12   2    5    5    9    6    9
25001    25173    99034    99035   1  3    1  .
4    5   12  13    4    6    3   12   2    5    5    9    6    9
25001    99034      0               0  1  3    1  .
.    .    .    .    .    .    .    .    .    .    .    .    .    .
25001    99035      0               0  2  3    2  .
.    .    .    .    .    .    .    .    .    .    .    .    .    .
25003    25003    25024    99016   1  3    1  2
4    5   11  13    .    .    .    .    4    5    7    7    .    .
.....................................................................
.....................................................................
39057    85007      0               0  2  3    2  1
.    .    .    .    .    .    .    .    .    .    .    .    .    .
39059    39004    85004    85005   2  3    2  2
3    4   11  12    3    6    .    .    .    .    8    8    .    .
39059    39059    85004    85005   1  3    1  2
4    6    7  12    .    .    7   11   4    5    .    .    6    9
39059    39060    85004    85005   1  3    1  2
3    4   11  12    3    6    4    7   3    3    8   10    6    7
39059    85004      0               0  1  3    1  1
.    .    .    .    .    .    .    .    .    .    .    .    .    .
39059    85005      0               0  2  3    2  .
.    .    .    .    .    .    .    .    .    .    .    .    .    .
```

Textbox 2. Part of the data file for the example in this chapter.

ables. The *function* parameters may appear anywhere in the parameter file, but they are processed immediately after the pedigree data are read, in the order that they appear. A function variable may be used just like a trait, phenotype, or covariate in the later SAGE analysis. Readers can consult the SAGE documentation for detail.

3.1.3. Marker Locus Description File

The marker locus description file and the trait locus description file (used for model-based linkage analysis) each follow the same format and contain records that define allele frequencies and marker phenotype to genotype mapping. For codominant markers, the mapping is unique and thus is not required to specify. The information (or data) for markers should be consistently included in the parameter file, data file, genome description file, and locus description file. **Textbox 3** shows part of the locus description file for the chapter example.

```
#Missing=Code # optionally, a missing value code may be included.
GATA69E12 # the first marker name
   3    =   0.3587217 # the allelic frequency for allele "3"
   4    =   0.2870398
   5    =   0.2383826
   2    =   0.0899924
   1    =   0.0103623
   6    =   0.0155013
;                     # the separator between markers
;
GATA88G05
  12    =   0.3067480
  13    =   0.2137845
  11    =   0.1800197
  15    =   0.0287466
..........................
..........................
GGAA20G04 # the last marker name
   6    =   0.1437366
   7    =   0.1141430
   9    =   0.3266727
   5    =   0.1076162
  10    =   0.0819375
   4    =   0.0402426
   8    =   0.1551106
   3    =   0.0222511 .
   2    =   0.0036844
  11    =   0.0036844
   1    =   0.0009208
;
;
```

Textbox 3. Marker locus description file.

3.1.4. Genome Description File

A genome description file describes the genomic region(s) used in some analysis that requires the order, and distance between, linked marker loci; for example, multipoint IBD computation as implemented in the SAGE program GENIBD. The between-marker distances, usually expressed in centimorgans, can be translated into recombination fraction using either the Haldane or Kosambi map function. The example genome file is given in **Textbox 4**.

3.1.5. IBD Sharing File

The IBD sharing file, generated by the SAGE program GENIBD, stores the probability distribution of allele-sharing IBD between pairs of individuals at specific locations, and can be used as an input file to programs such as SIBPAL. We will describe the file in the later implementation of GENIBD.

```
Genome # a user can specify the genome name and mapping function here
{
#chromosome2
region=chr02 # the region name
{
marker="GATA69E12"  # marker name
distance=12.0       # between-marker distance in centimorgans
marker="GATA88G05"
distance=11.0
marker="GATA176C01"
distance=11.0
marker="GATA4E11"
distance=7.4
marker="GATA27A12"
distance=13.0
marker="GATA4D07"
distance=6.9
marker="GGAA20G04"
}
}
```

Textbox 4. Genome description file.

3.2. Data Checking

Data checking and error corrections are essential prior to performing adequate and accurate genetic data analysis, especially for large-scale model-free linkage analysis, in which massive pedigree data are recruited. It is often the case that these data pre-processing jobs can take significant proportion of the time for performing a complete large-scale genetic analysis. SAGE provides several powerful programs, described as follows, to check and to identify potential errors and inconsistencies inherent in the studied pedigree data.

3.2.1. PEDINFO for Descriptive Statistic on Pedigree Structure

PEDINFO is often the first program to run, and provides many useful descriptive statistics on pedigree structure including means, variances, and histograms of family sibship and pedigree size, and counts of each type of relative pairs. Statistics based on trait phenotypic status (limited to traits not having missing values) can also be obtained. The below is the program block used in this example. The option "each_pedigree" allows calculating statistics on a pedigree-by-pedigree basis and the option "suppress_general" specifies suppression of output for nontrait statistics.

```
pedinfo, out=pedinfo_example.out
{
#each_pedigree=true
#suppress_general=true
}
```

PEDINFO requires two input file (the parameter file including the PEDINFO block and pedigree data file) to run, either interactively using the SAGE GUI or typing on a common line in UNIX or DOS. **Textbox 5** gives the PEDINFO output, the descriptive statistics for pedigrees in the example. The inheritance vector bits statistic is the value of 2n-f maximized over constitute pedigrees, where n is the number of nonfounders and f is the number of founders in each constituent pedigree. It is useful to evaluate whether it is feasible to run certain types of multipoint analysis algorithms on a given pedigree. Several useful statistics also provide the user the information for potential data errors. Information for "Individuals with Multiple Mates" suggests either truly multiple marriages or a data error. Likewise, "Singleton" individuals are either a fact, such as marry-ins without any children (thus not useful for pedigree data analysis), or a data error. PEDINFO can also identify a list of problematic family structures, which is described in detail in the SAGE documentation.

3.2.2. FREQ Analysis for Obtaining Unbiased and Accurate Marker Allelic Frequencies

It is known that misspecification of marker allelic frequencies can seriously bias both model-free and model-based linkage analysis. The true allelic frequencies of markers represent the population frequencies that the collected pedigrees refer to and can be estimated (or obtained) from one of the following: (1) the previous literature, (2) public databases, (3) genotyping population-based samples, (4) the recruited pedigree data by maximum likelihood methods. FREQ is such a program that estimates allele frequencies from marker data among related individuals with known pedigree structure, and generates marker locus description files needed by GENIBD and other SAGE programs. For co-dominant markers, FREQ requires two input files (the parameter file and the data file) to run. The below is the block for FREQ analysis for the example:

```
freq, out=freq_example.out
{
#skip_mle=true #Specify whether to skip ML computation of
allele frequencies
}
```

The option "skip_mle" allows a user to choose the method of estimating marker allelic frequencies. If the value is "true," FREQ will use the Initial Frequencies Estimator to compute allele frequencies using only founders and singletons or using other individuals or combined by a founder-weight parameter. In the Maximum Likelihood Estimator (mle), the likelihood for the data at each marker in the whole sample is numerically maximized over possible allele

```
                              pedinfo_example.out
S.A.G.E. v5.0 -- PEDINFO
COPYRIGHT (C) 2004 CASE WESTERN RESERVE UNIVERSITY

File generated on : Tue Jul 19 14:34:46 2005


|===================================================================================|
|                    General Statistics: All Pedigrees                              |
|===================================================================================|
|              | Count| Mean Size +/- Std. Dev. (     Min.,      Max.)              |
|-----------------------------------------------------------------------------------|
| Pedigrees    |   409|     4.84 +/-      2.36 (        3,        43)               |
|===================================================================================|
| Generation Statistics|| Nuc  Family Statistics ||  Inh  Vector Bit Stats           |
| # of Gens  | # of Peds|| # of Nuc Fams |# of Peds||   # of Bits  |# of Peds         |
|-----------------------------------------------------------------------------------|
|          2|       399||    0 -      2|     404||    0 -      2|           232      |
|          3|         9||    3 -      4|       4||    3 -      4|           107      |
|          4|         0||    5 -      8|       0||    5 -      8|            54      |
|          5|         1||    9 -     16|       1||    9 -     16|            14      |
|           |          ||             |        ||   17 -     32|             1      |
|           |          ||             |        ||   33 -     64|             1      |
|===================================================================================|
|              | Count| Mean Size +/- Std. Dev. (     Min.,      Max.)              |
|-----------------------------------------------------------------------------------|
| Sibships     |   444|     2.53 +/-      1.21 (        1,        10)               |
|===================================================================================|
| Constituent  |         || Marriage  |          ||                  |               |
| Pedigrees    |     409|| Rings     |         0|| Loops            |            0   |
|===================================================================================|
| Pairs        |           Count|| Individuals         |            Count            |
|-----------------------------------------------------------------------------------|
| Parent/off   |            2250|| Male                |             1124            |
| Sib/Sib      |            1189|| Female              |              854            |
| Sis/Sis      |             240|| Unknown             |                0            |
| Bro/Bro      |             430||             Total   |             1978            |
| Bro/Sis      |             519||                     |                            |
| Grandp.      |             104|| Founder             |              853            |
| Avunc.       |             146|| Non-founder         |             1125            |
| Half Sib     |              41|| Singleton           |                0            |
| Cousin       |             158||             Total   |             1978            |
|===================================================================================|
|                     Individuals with Multiple Mates                               |
| (Pedigree, Individual)   Mates                                                    |
|-----------------------------------------------------------------------------------|
| (25063, 99238)        99237, 99241                                                |
| (25265, 99216)        99220, 99219                                                |
| (25396, 99317)        99318, 99316                                                |
| (25451, 99320)        99319, 99323                                                |
| (25569, 99434)        99436, 99435                                                |
| (28253, 96061)        96060, 77001                                                |
| (28263, 28230)        96082, 77002                                                |
| (28265, 96084)        96083, 96085                                                |
| (28275, 96071)        77003, 96070                                                |
| (29085, 29006)        77004, 95036                                                |
| (36065, 88013)        88014, 77005                                                |
|===================================================================================|
|                     Consanguineous Mating Pairs                                   |
| none                                                                              |
|===================================================================================|
```

Textbox 5. PEDINFO output: the descriptive statistics for pedigrees in the example.

frequencies to obtain the maximum likelihood estimates for that marker. Like most of SAGE programs, FREQ produces several output files. For the chapter example, three files are generated: "freq.inf" containing informational diagnostic messages; "freq_example.out.out" containing the detailed tables of analysis options and results, including the standard error for each maximum likelihood frequency estimate; and "freq_example.out.loc," the locus description file, part of which is shown in **Textbox 3**.

3.2.3. RELTEST for Correcting Any Familial Relationship Error

Familial relationship errors can often occur in a large sample of pedigrees owing to a variety of reasons. RELTEST analysis, based on a Markov process model of allele sharing along chromosomes, provides a way to identify and correct any familial relationship error using genome-wide marker data. The program currently performs analyses to classify putative sib pairs, putative half sib pairs, putative parent–offspring pairs, and putative marital pairs into five different pairs: MZ twin pairs, full sib pairs, half sib pairs, parent–offspring pairs, and unrelated pairs. The probability of misclassification depends on the total length of the genotyped genome provided and overall marker informativeness. The misclassification rates are minimal when at least half the genome is genotyped and analyzed using microsatellite markers that are at most 20 cM apart. Therefore, we choose not to demonstrate this analysis because this example only uses seven markers on one chromosome. Readers can consult with the SAGE documentation for the detail for performing this analysis. However, for the chapter example, the GeneGuest pedigrees are the remaining pedigrees after correction of some familial relationship errors in 58 pedigrees, and removal of 27 pedigrees with uncorrectable errors.

3.2.4. MARKERINFO for Checking Any Mendelian Inconsistencies of Marker Data

Checking any Mendelian inconsistencies in marker data is a routine task in model-based linkage analysis, and can be performed using the LINKAGE program UNKNOWN (*see* Chapter 5). The SAGE package also provides a similar module, called MARKERINFO. Although this data-checking is not a "standard" for model-free linkage analysis, thoroughly checking the pedigree data analyzed is highly recommended. Below is the parameter block for MARKERINFO analysis corresponding to the chapter example:

```
markerinfo, out=markerinfor_example.out
{
#sample_id="the name of a field in the pedigree file"
#consistent_out="true or false for outputting inconsistency
symbol []"
}
```

Two options within the block control the contents of the output file. MARKERINFO requires the parameter file and the pedigree data file to run, and then generates two output files: one file contains informational diagnostic messages, and the other is the analysis output file (i.e., markerinfor_ example.out). Part of the file is shown in **Textbox 6**.

Part 1 of this output file gives the statistics for number of inconsistencies per pedigree or per marker and Part 2 gives the detailed information for inconsistencies. Two examples of Mendelian inconsistencies are shown.

We have now introduced several SAGE programs for data checking and error corrections. It should be noted that there is no optimal sequence(s) of programs to implement this job. Whether a program can produce the most accurate results depends, to some extent, on the results from other programs. For example, RELTEST checks familial relationships by assuming no error in marker data, whereas MARKERINFO checks for Mendelian inconsistencies in marker data by assuming no pedigree relationship errors. Therefore, it usually requires several cycles between these programs or reliance one's basic data-management skills to reduce potential data errors to a minimum.

3.3. Linkage Analysis

3.3.1. GENIBD for Computing IBD Data for Linkage Analysis

GENIBD provides three methods of generating IBD sharing: the single-marker IBD analysis or multipoint IBD analysis, controlled by "ibd_mode" in the GENIBD block as shown below, or the simulation IBD analysis (specified using the statement "use_simulation"). GENIBD also provides the option of splitting a large pedigree into nuclear families before processing.

```
GENIBD, out=ibd_example.out
{
title="SP" # specify title of the run
ibd_mode="singlepoint" # either singlepoint or multipoint
region=chr02 # the region in genomic description file to be run
#scan_type=intervals #default value is "markers"
#distance=2.0
use_simulation=false # allow simulation on large pedigrees
#split_pedigrees=yes # option to split large pedigrees
}
```

GENIBD requires three files (parameter file, pedigree data file, and marker locus description file) for computing single-point IBD profiles, and an additional file (genome description file) to run multipoint IBD computations. To execute this program (e.g., for the chapter example), either use the SAGE GUI (**Fig. 3**) or type on a command line in the supported UNIX or DOS platforms:

> **genibd Parchr02_MP.par Chr02_rev_MP.DAT freq_example.out.loc**

The resulting output files (GENIBD.inf, genome.inf and ibd_example.out. REGION.ibd) list, at each location, the probability of each pair sharing 0 or 2

```
S.A.G.E. v5.0 -- MARKERINFO
COPYRIGHT (C) 2004 CASE WESTERN RESERVE UNIVERSITY
File generated on : Tue Jul 19 14:42:51 2005
======================================================================
    Markerinfo Analysis Output
======================================================================
----------------------------------------------------------------------
    Part 1: Number of Inconsistencies per pedigree/marker
----------------------------------------------------------------------
======================================================================
                                         Number of Markers
Pedigree                        Incon.     with Data        Total
----------                      ------    -------------    ----------
25042                              1             7              7
25455                              1             7              7
.......................................................................
36065                              1             7              7
======================================================================
======================================================================
                                         Number of Pedigrees
Marker                          Incon.     with Data        Total
----------                      ------    -------------    ----------
GGAA20G04                          4            363            409
GATA88G05                          3            368            409
GATA4D07                           3            361            409
GATA69E12                          1            373            409
======================================================================
----------------------------------------------------------------------
    Part 2: Inconsistencies
----------------------------------------------------------------------
======================================================================
Table 1 with Marker  GGAA20G04  GATA88G05  GATA4D07
======================================================================
Pedigree    Individual          GGAA20G04      GATA88G05      GATA4D07
----------  ----------          ----------     ----------     ----------
25042       99059    Mother                                     ./.
25042       99058    Father                                     ./.
25042       25218                                               9/6
25042       25175                                               9/9
25042       25042                                               7/8
.......................................................................
======================================================================
======================================================================
Table 2 with Marker  GATA69E12
======================================================================
Pedigree    Individual          GATA69E12
----------  ----------          ----------
36062       36010    Mother     3/3
36062       88009    Father     ./.
36062       36063
36062       36062               4/2
36062       36009
======================================================================
```

Textbox 6. MARKERINFO output for Mendelian inconsistency information on markers.

alleles IBD, and the difference between the paternal and maternal probability of sharing 1 allele IBD, conditional as a condition of the marker data available. The file "ibd_example.out.REGION.ibd" can then be read into other programs (e.g., SIBPAL) for analysis. On the first line of the IBD data file, the warning "Do NOT edit!" is given to ensure that this input file is read correctly by other SAGE programs. Thus, we choose not to show the contents of this file here, as no user interference with this file is required.

3.3.2. SIBPAL for Evaluating Model-Free Linkage Evidence

Once the pedigree data file is preprocessed and the IBD data are computed, performing H-E sib-pair regression using the SAGE program SIBPAL is straightforward. This program models trait data from full and half sib pairs as a function of marker IBD. Available options can use both single- and multipoint IBD, and allow for both binary and continuous traits due to multiple genetic loci, including epistatic interactions, and covariate effects. For a demonstration, we perform a single-point regression using seven markers in the chapter example. Here is the corresponding parameter

```
trait_regression, out=HE_example.out
{
#regression_method=w2 # one of six types of dependent variable
trait=MI # the trait used as the dependent variable
covariate=race # covariate 1
covariate=gender # covariate 2
#compute_empirical_pvalues=true,threshold
="0.00074",max_replicates=100000
#subset="the indicator for using only subset of the data"
}
```

The "trait_regression" block is a subblock of the sibpal block, which can also include the subblock "mean_test" to perform a nonparametric test of mean IBD sharing. In the current SAGE version, SIBPAL allows a total of six definitions (product as the default) of the dependent variable, specified by the statement "regression_method," which include (1) squared trait difference; (2) squared mean-corrected trait sum; (3) mean-corrected cross-product; and (4) three weighted combinations of (1) and (2). SIBPAL also allows the inclusion of several definitions (product as the default) of covariates to perform multiple regression. For a small-sized pedigree sample and genome-wide linkage analysis, obtaining a robust p value for linkage evidence can be critical. Thus, SIBPAL provides a solution for estimating an empirical p value by permutations, specified by "compute_empirical_pvalues." A user can define the threshold for an asymptotic p value (say, 0.00074) to be re-computed using a certain number of permutations (e.g., 100,000). The statement "subset" is useful for heterogeneous samples (e.g., mixture of different races) and can stratify the sample into more homogeneous subsets.

SIBPAL requires three files to run, and produces up to three files (sibpal.inf, means.out, and traits.out). The modified H-E sib-pair regression for the chapter example can be performed by typing at a command line:

>**sibpal Parchr02_MP.par Chr02_rev_MP.DAT ibd_example.out. REGION.ibd**

It is recommended that the user check the information file (sibpal.inf) for warning and error messages before examining the results of any run of the program. The file "HE_example.out.out" for this example is shown in **Textbox 7**, which contains the results of the regression parameter corresponding to the total genetic variance (additive plus dominant), its standard error and nominal *p* value of an asymptotic t-test described already.

3.4. Alternative Approaches and Programs for Linkage Analysis of Complex Traits

3.4.1. Logarithm of the Odds Score Approaches

The first approach is to set the penetrance of the disease gene close to zero, and the sporadic risk (i.e., the risk among disease-gene noncarriers) much closer to zero. This modeling scheme uses information from the affected individuals. The unaffected individuals are almost equally likely to be either carriers or noncarriers, and thus are uninformative for the linkage analysis. Strictly speaking, this approach is not model-free because a genetic model is assumed (e.g., dominant or recessive). Nevertheless, in 1989, Risch et al. *(19)* performed simulation studies and showed that the approach provided a good preliminary test for linkage. A second approach for applying logarithm of the odds (lod) score methods to complex traits is the mod score approach *(20)*, in which the lod score is maximized over both the penetrance and the recombination fraction. This method is included in the SAGE module MLOD.

3.4.2. Other Methods and Software for Analyzing Sib-Pair and Sibship Data

Many tests (e.g., ref. *21*) based on IBD (or IBS) means are simple enough to be analyzed using a standard statistical package if the IBD statistic can be determined with certainty. For complicated pedigree likelihood computations, a list of programs can be found in the Rockefeller site for linkage programs (e.g., MAPMAKER/SIBS *[22]*, SimWalk *[23]*) (http://linkage.rockefeller.edu/).

3.4.3. Affected Only Analysis

This analysis is useful for late-onset cardiovascular diseases or in cases in which the age at onset cannot be well specified. In these cases, phenotypic

```
S.A.G.E. v5.0 -- SIBPAL
COPYRIGHT (C) 2004 CASE WESTERN RESERVE UNIVERSITY
File generated on : Tue Jul 19 14:51:02 2005
 #######################################################
 #                                                     #
 #  ANALYSIS OF FULL SIB COVARIANCE: Single regression #
 #                                                     #
 #   Using all markers since none were specified.      #
 #                                                     #
 #######################################################

Regression for binary trait                            'MI'.
Dependent variable         Mean-corrected trait cross-product
Number of full sib pairs                      =       315
Independent
variates:
Marker,
Covariate or                                          Nominal
Interaction    Pairs  Parameter    Estimate  Std Error  P-value
-------------- -----  -----------  --------- ---------- ---------
race           315    Cov,prod      -0.0050    0.0229  8.289e-01
gender         315    Cov,prod      -0.0135    0.0175  4.403e-01
gender         315    Cov,prod      -0.0135    0.0175  4.403e-01
race           315    Cov,prod      -0.0050    0.0229  8.289e-01
GATA69E12      285    (A+D)GenVar    0.0093    0.0452  4.189e-01
race           285    Cov,prod      -0.0043    0.0260  8.691e-01
gender         285    Cov,prod      -0.0161    0.0187  3.899e-01
GATA88G05      270    (A+D)GenVar    0.0842    0.0384  1.453e-02
race           270    Cov,prod      -0.0022    0.0291  9.388e-01
gender         270    Cov,prod      -0.0245    0.0186  1.886e-01
GATA176C01     223    (A+D)GenVar    0.0061    0.0558  4.567e-01
race           223    Cov,prod      -0.0028    0.0195  8.862e-01
gender         223    Cov,prod       0.0140    0.0206  4.977e-01
GATA4E11       248    (A+D)GenVar    0.0264    0.0442  2.759e-01
race           248    Cov,prod      -0.0037    0.0473  9.378e-01
gender         248    Cov,prod      -0.0247    0.0191  1.982e-01
GATA27A12      267    (A+D)GenVar    0.1018    0.0439  1.059e-02
race           267    Cov,prod      -0.0013    0.0284  9.624e-01
gender         267    Cov,prod       0.0078    0.0189  6.802e-01
GATA4D07       257    (A+D)GenVar    0.0769    0.0467  5.047e-02
race           257    Cov,prod      -0.0018    0.0211  9.335e-01
gender         257    Cov,prod      -0.0219    0.0188  2.452e-01
GGAA20G04      247    (A+D)GenVar   -0.0449    0.0516  8.076e-01
race           247    Cov,prod      -0.0016    0.0217  9.428e-01
gender         247    Cov,prod       0.0073    0.0187  6.976e-01
=================================================================
```

Textbox 7. SIBPAL output for Haseman-Elston sibpair regression.

evaluations for affected individuals are much more accurate than for "normal" individuals. Several methods involving parametric (e.g., the SAGE program LODPAL [24]), or nonparametric tests (e.g., Affected Pedigree Member

[APM] *[25]*, SimIBD analysis *[26]*, Non-Parametric Linkage [NPL] *[27]*, the Weighted Pairwise Correlation [WPC] *[28]*) have been developed.

3.4.4. Variance Component Methods

SOLAR *(29)* is a flexible and extensive software package for genetic variance components analysis, including linkage analysis, quantitative genetic analysis, and covariate screening. Recently, we have witnessed rapidly increasing application of the method in the model-free linkage analysis.

Acknowledgments

This work was supported by the National Institutes of Health (NIH) grants R01 HL65630, R01 HL66251, P50 HL77107, and an American Heart Association Established Investigator award (to Q.K.W.). Some of the results of this chapter were obtained using the program package SAGE, which is supported by a US Public Health Service Resource Grant (RR03655) from the National Center for Research Resources.

Further Reading

1. Haseman and Elston, "The investigation of linkage between a quantitative trait and a marker locus" *(4)*: in this seminal paper, the authors provided the basic theory and mathematical derivations to relate the genetic similarity of a sib pair with their phenotypic similarity. This theoretical paper established the basis for various IBD-based linkage analysis approaches.
2. Elston et al., "Haseman and Elston revisited" *(18)*: this paper describes the major advances for sib-pair-based linkage analysis, resulting from recent methodological investigations by numerous genetic epidemiologists. The authors focused on extensions of the original H-E regression in three aspects: (1) additional definitions of the dependent variable; (2) multivariate modeling; and (3) accommodation of more involved genetic hypothesis (e.g., epistatic interactions); all of which have also been incorporated into the current SAGE version.
3. SAGE developers, "SAGE Version 5.0 User Reference Manual" *(11)*: This volume (354 pages) contains detailed user's guides for 14 modules for statistical analysis of genetic data.

References

1. Morton, N. E. (1955) Sequential tests for the detection of linkage. *Am. J. Hum. Genet.* **7,** 277–318.
2. Wang, Q., Rao, S., and Topol, E. J. (2004) Reply to newton-cheh et al. *Am. J. Hum. Genet.* **75,** 152–154.
3. Farrer, L. A. and Cupples, L. A. (1998) 5. Determining the genetic component of a disease, in *Approaches to Gene Mapping in Complex Human Diseases,* (Haines, J. L. and Pericak-Vance, M. A. eds.), Wiley-Liss, New York, pp. 93–129.

 4. Haseman, J. K. and Elston, R. C. (1972) The investigation of linkage between a quantitative trait and a marker locus. *Behav. Genet.* **2,** 3–19.
 5. Amos, C. I. and Elston, R. C. (1989) Robust methods for the detection of genetic linkage for quantitative data from pedigrees. *Genet. Epidemiol.* **6,** 349–360.
 6. Wright, F. A. (1997) The phenotypic difference discards sib-pair QTL linkage information. *Am. J. Hum. Genet.* **60,** 740–742.
 7. Fulker, D. W. and Cherny, S. S. (1996) An improved multipoint sib-pair analysis of quantitative traits. *Behav. Genet.* **26,** 527–532.
 8. Amos, C. I., Krushkal, J., Thiel, T. J., et al. (1997) Comparison of model-free linkage mapping strategies for the study of a complex trait. *Genet. Epidemiol.* **14,** 743–748.
 9. Single, R. M. and Finch, S. J. (1995) Gain in efficiency from using generalized least squares in the Haseman-Elston test. *Genet. Epidemiol.* **12,** 889–894.
10. Karunaratne, P. M. and Elston, R. C. (1998) A multivariate logistic model (MLM) for analyzing binary family data. *Am. J. Med. Genet.* **76,** 428–437.
11. SAGE (2004) *SAGE Version 5.0. User Reference Manual,* Department of Epidemiology and Biostatistics, Case Western Reserve University, Cleveland, OH.
12. Bonney, G. E. (1986) Regressive logistic models for familial disease and other binary traits. *Biometrics* **42,** 611–625.
13. Hanson, R. L., Elston, R. C., Pettitt, D. J., Bennett, P. H., and Knowler, W. C. (1995) Segregation analysis of non-insulin-dependent diabetes mellitus in Pima Indians: evidence for a major-gene effect. *Am. J. Hum. Genet.* **57,** 160–170.
14. Elston, R. C. (1981) Segregation analysis. *Adv. Hum. Genet.* **11,** 63–120, 372–123.
15. Olson, J. M. (1999) Relationship estimation by Markov-process models in a sib-pair linkage study. *Am. J. Hum. Genet.* **64,** 1464–1472.
16. Topol, E. J., McCarthy, J., Gabriel, S., et al. (2001) Single nucleotide polymorphisms in multiple novel thrombospondin genes may be associated with familial premature myocardial infarction. *Circulation* **104,** 2641–2644.
17. Wang, Q., Rao, S., Shen, G. Q., et al. (2004) Premature myocardial infarction novel susceptibility locus on chromosome 1P34-36 identified by genomewide linkage analysis. *Am. J. Hum. Genet.* **74,** 262–271.
18. Elston, R. C., Buxbaum, S., Jacobs, K. B., and Olson, J. M. (2000) Haseman and Elston revisited. *Genet. Epidemiol.* **19,** 1–17.
19. Risch, N., Claus, E., and Giuffra, L. (1989) Linkage and mode of inheritance in complex traits. *Prog. Clin. Biol. Res.* **329,** 183–188.
20. Hodge, S. E. and Elston, R. C. (1994) Lods, wrods, and mods: the interpretation of lod scores calculated under different models. *Genet. Epidemiol.* **11,** 329–342.
21. Lange, K. (1986) The affected sib-pair method using identity by state relations. *Am. J. Hum. Genet.* **39,** 148–150.
22. Kruglyak, L. and Lander, E. S. (1995) Complete multipoint sib-pair analysis of qualitative and quantitative traits. *Am. J. Hum. Genet.* **57,** 439–454.
23. Sobel, E. and Lange, K. (1996) Descent graphs in pedigree analysis: applications to haplotyping, location scores, and marker-sharing statistics. *Am. J. Hum. Genet.* **58,** 1323–1337.

24. Olson, J. M. (1999) A general conditional-logistic model for affected-relative-pair linkage studies. *Am. J. Hum. Genet.* **65,** 1760–1769.
25. Weeks, D. E. and Lange, K. (1988) The affected-pedigree-member method of linkage analysis. *Am. J. Hum. Genet.* **42,** 315–326.
26. Davis, S., Schroeder, M., Goldin, L. R., and Weeks, D. E. (1996) Nonparametric simulation-based statistics for detecting linkage in general pedigrees. *Am. J. Hum. Genet.* **58,** 867–880.
27. Kruglyak, L., Daly, M. J., Reeve-Daly, M. P., and Lander, E. S. (1996) Parametric and nonparametric linkage analysis: a unified multipoint approach. *Am. J. Hum. Genet.* **58,** 1347–1363.
28. Commenges, D. (1994) Robust genetic linkage analysis based on a score test of homogeneity: the weighted pairwise correlation statistic. *Genet. Epidemiol.* **11,** 189–200.
29. Almasy, L. and Blangero, J. (1998) Multipoint quantitative-trait linkage analysis in general pedigrees. *Am. J. Hum. Genet.* **62,** 1198–1211.

7

Linkage Analysis for Complex Diseases Using Variance Component Analysis

SOLAR

Ulrich Broeckel, Karen Maresso, and Lisa J. Martin

Summary

Variance component linkage analysis has become one of the most popular tools for the analysis of polygenic phenotypes. In particular for cardiovascular disease, such as coronary artery disease and myocardial infarction, variance component analysis holds some unique advantages. This analysis approach is versatile, affording the user the ability to incorporate the interplay between risk factors, genetic susceptibility, the effect of environmental factors, or the joint analysis of multiple phenotypes in the analysis. In this chapter, we present as an introduction the statistical background of variance component analysis as implemented in the genetic analysis package SOLAR.

Key Words: Cardiovascular disease; variance component analysis; gene–environment analysis; linkage analysis; polygenic disease; quantitative trait locus; QTL.

1. Introduction

Coronary artery disease (CAD) and myocardial infarction (MI) are the leading causes of death in both men and women of all races *(1)*. Cardiovascular risk factors, such as diabetes mellitus, arterial hypertension, or hypercholesterolemia, contribute significantly to the development of the disease. Although these risk factors by themselves are, in part, under genetic control, a positive family history is an additional important independent predictor *(2,3)*. Given the complex interaction and interdependence between risk factor and disease susceptibility, the genetic analysis aiming to improve our understanding of the underlying genetic basis of CAD therefore poses some significant challenges. Ultimately, the goal of a comprehensive analysis would be to incorporate our

From: *Methods in Molecular Medicine, Vol. 128: Cardiovascular Disease; Methods and Protocols; Volume 1*
Edited by: Q. Wang © Humana Press Inc., Totowa, NJ

initial understanding of the disease etiology and risk factor contribution to the disease. At the same time, the estimation of the interrelation with regard to the complex phenotypic pattern of CAD as well as the risk factors can give additional insights in the underlying genetic makeup of the disease process. Variance component analysis represents a versatile approach, and over the years the theoretical background has been developed to address, on a statistical and analytical level, some of the above-raised issues. This chapter will focus on some of the advanced features and analysis procedures that have been incorporated in the genetic linkage analysis software package Sequential Oligogenic Linkage Analysis Routine (SOLAR), in particular as they relate to gene–environment interactions.

2. Methods

2.1. Variance Component Analysis

2.1.1. Polygenic Analysis

In the variance components method, the phenotype of an individual is modeled as a linear function and given by the equation:

$$Y_i = \mu + \beta_j v_{ij} + g_i + e_i \tag{1}$$

where μ is the mean of the trait in males, β_j is the regression coefficient of the jth covariate, n_{ij} is the value of the jth covariate in the ith individual, and g_i and e_i represent the random deviations from μ for the ith individual that are attributable to additive genetic effects and unmeasured environmental effects, respectively (4). The effects of g_i and e_i are assumed to be uncorrelated with one another and normally distributed with mean 0 and variances σ_g^2 and σ_e^2. Given this linear relationship, the covariance between a set of relative pairs is a function of the additive genetic variance and the random environmental variance.

To permit the analysis of arbitrary pedigree structures, a structuring matrix is multiplied by each of the variances. The structuring matrix for the additive genetic variance is a matrix of kinship coefficients, whereas the structuring matrix for the environmental variance is an identity matrix (diagonal elements are ones and the rest of the elements are zeros), permitting unique environments for each individual.

From this model, the additive genetic and random environmental components of variation can be estimated given the variance–covariance matrix and the kinship coefficients. p Values for the heritability calculations are obtained by likelihood ratio tests, in which the likelihood of a model is estimated and compared with the likelihood of a model in which the heritability is constrained to zero. Twice the difference in these log-likelihoods is asymptotically distributed as a one-half:one-half mixture of a χ^2 variable with one degree of freedom and a point mass at zero *(5)*.

Although there are various methods of estimating polygenic inheritance, the generalized variance component method has several advantages over other approaches *(4)*. Specifically, this method is powerful and flexible. The power of the variance component method can be attributed to three major factors: minimization of nongenetic variation, utilization of population variance, and the ability to use arbitrary pedigree structures *(6–9)*. The flexibility of the variance components method is attributed to its ability to handle pedigrees of arbitrary size and complexity, allowing for incorporation of non-Mendelian effects such as genotype by environment interaction, epistasis, threshold models, pleiotropy, multivariate analyses, and mitochondrial inheritance and oligogenic analyses *(7,10–13)*.

2.1.2. Linkage Analysis

The variance component linkage method is based on the theory that by partitioning out nongenetic variation, characterization of genetic effects is simplified *(14,15)*. The goal is to determine whether genetic variation at a specific marker locus can explain the variation in the phenotype *(15)*. When genes are linked, phenotypic variability owing to a specific marker locus is a function of the distance between the marker gene and the gene causing the trait (recombination fraction) and the relationship between individuals. When genes are unlinked, the genetic variance component depends only on the relationship between individuals *(14)*.

To estimate linkage, the variance component method examines how the phenotypes of related individuals co-vary given the relationship between the individuals and the proportion of genes shared identical-by-descent (IBD) at a specific marker locus *(16)*. To test for linkage, a LOD score, the ratio of the likelihood of a linkage model to basic polygenic model with no linkage, is calculated. Therefore, for each marker, a logarithm of the odds (lod) score is calculated to test its probability of being linked with a trait.

2.1.3. Multipoint Variance Component Analysis in SOLAR

Multipoint variance component linkage analysis is a simple extension of basic quantitative genetic theory. In this method, the genetic variance attributable to the region of a specific genetic marker is estimated by specifying the expected genetic covariances between arbitrary relatives as a function of the IBD relationships at a quantitative trait locus (QTL) *(4)*. Given this, the covariance matrix, Ω, is

$$\Omega = \Sigma \hat{\Pi}_i \, \sigma_{qi}^2 + 2\Phi\sigma_g^2 + I\sigma_e^2$$

where σ_{qi}^2 is the additive genetic variance due to the ith QTL, $\hat{\Pi}_i$ is a matrix whose elements $\hat{\Pi}_{ijk}$ provide the predicted proportion of genes that individuals j and k share IBD at a QTL that is linked to a marker locus, σ_g^2 is the genetic variance due to residual additive genetic factors, Φ is the kinship matrix, σ_e^2 is the variance due to individual specific environmental effects, and I is the identity matrix.

$\hat{\Pi}$ is a function of the IBD matrix for genetic marker(s) and a matrix of correlations between the proportions of genes IBD at the marker and at the QTL and is defined as

$$\hat{\Pi}_i = 2\Phi + \mathbf{B}(r,\theta) \; \left(\hat{\Pi}_m - 2\Phi\right) \tag{3}$$

where $\hat{\Pi}_i$ is a matrix whose elements provide the predicted proportion of genes that a pair of individuals share IBD at a QTL that is linked to a genetic marker and is a function of the estimated IBD matrix for a genetic marker, $\hat{\Pi}_m$, and a matrix of correlations, B, between the proportions of genes IBD at the marker and the QTL. θ is the recombination frequency between marker locus m and QTLi, and the elements $b_{ij} = \rho(\pi_i, \pi_m \,|\, r,\theta)$ are the correlations between IBD probabilities, where r denotes the rth type of kinship relationship.

In SOLAR, the IBD matrix is a multipoint IBD (MIBD) matrix, which utilizes marker information across the chromosome, such that the markers closest to the location have the strongest impact for a specific point. The calculation of MIBDs for arbitrary pedigree structures requires correlation functions $\left[\rho(\pi_i, \pi_j \,|\, r,\theta)\right]$ for all possible relative pairs *(4)*. These equations can be used to provide the expected IBD correlation between genotyped marker loci and the estimated multipoint chromosomal locations, $\hat{\pi}$. The correlation in the proportion of alleles shared IBD by a relative pair over some chromosomal distance can be expressed by

$$\rho(\pi_1, \pi_2 \,|\, r,\theta) = \frac{Cov(\pi_1, \pi_2)}{\sigma(\pi_1)\sigma(\pi_2)}$$

where $Cov(\pi_1, \pi_2)$ is the covariance of the IBD allele sharing between locus 1 (the genotyped marker) and locus 2 (the arbitrary chromosomal location at which IBD sharing is being estimated), and $\sigma(\pi_1)$ and $\sigma(\pi_2)$ are the expected standard deviations in IBD allele sharing at the two loci.

To estimate MIBD probabilities, Blangero et al. *(4,17)* use the generalized regression-based averaging method of Fulker et al. *(18)*. For any pair of individuals of relationship, r, they calculate the vector of regression coefficients (β_r) on the available estimated marker-specific $\hat{\pi}_z$ vectors that predict π , where   refers to chromosomal location *(4)*. Each chromosome's MIBDs are calculated independent of the other chromosomes. β_r is defined by the standard regression equation:

$$\beta_r = \mathbf{V}(\hat{\pi}_z)^{-1} Cov(\hat{\pi}_z, \pi)$$

where β_r is a vector of *n* regression coefficients, $\mathbf{V}(\hat{\pi}_z)$ is the $n \times n$ covariance matrix of the marker IBD probabilities, and $Cov(\hat{\pi}_z, \pi)$ is a vector of the expected covariances between the marker IBD probabilities and those at the chromosomal location . The elements of $\mathbf{V}(\hat{\pi})$ are determined by the genetic distances between the markers, the function of the correlation coefficients for IBD allele sharing in relative pairs, and the empirical variances of the $\hat{\pi}_i$.

Once obtained, the β_r vector is used to estimate the proportion of alleles shared IBD for a particular chromosomal location for the *ij*th pair of relatives by

$$\hat{\pi}_{lij} = 2\phi_r + \beta_r' \left(\hat{\pi} - \bar{\hat{\pi}} \right)$$

The MIBDs can then be used in linkage analysis routines to estimate linkage of a phenotype with a chromosomal region.

In summary, an individual's phenotype is a function of three components: a set of QTL effects, an additive polygenic effect, and a random environmental deviation. As demonstrated previously, the covariance matrix between two individuals is a function of the relationship between the variance attributable to the QTL and the genes shared IBD at that QTL, the additive variance and the kinship, and the environmental variance and the identity matrix. By partitioning the covariance into specific components, we are then able to test hypotheses of linkage on the premise that we can accurately estimate the different parameters of covariance.

2.2. Gene–Environment Analysis

Of particular interest for the analysis of disease susceptibility related to CAD and MI is the examination of how environmental factors might interact with disease and disease susceptibility genes. Based on epidemiological and experimental studies, it is accepted that the underlying disease susceptibility for cardiovascular diseases depends significantly on the risk factor profile. Therefore, analyses that can incorporate gene-by-environment (G×E) analyses should be more powerful and provide a disease-appropriate analysis approach. In that framework, a number of methods have been developed.

Regardless of the approach, the test for G×E interactions is based on hypotheses concerning the nature of the variance–covariance relationship of a trait between relative pairs under different environments *(19–21)*. The expected genetic covariance between a pair of relatives consisting of an individual with environment 1 and an individual with environment 2 is defined as

$$\mathrm{COV}\left(G_{E1}, G_{E2}\right) = 2\phi\ \rho_{G(E1,E2)}\ \sigma_{gE1}\ \sigma_{gE2}$$

where ϕ is the coefficient of kinship between the two individuals, $\rho_{G(E1,E2)}$ is the genetic correlation between the expressions of the trait in the two groups, and σ_{gE1} and σ_{gE2} are the genetic standard deviations for environment 1 and environment 2, respectively.

In the absence of G×E status interaction (i.e., the null hypothesis), the genetic correlation between relatives for a trait measured in environment 1 and environment 2 should be one $[\rho_{G(E1,E2)} = 1.0]$ and the genetic variances of the two groups should be equal (i.e., $\sigma_{gE1} = \sigma_{gE2}$) *(20,22)*. Conversely, if there is G×E interaction, the genetic correlation between the groups $[\rho_{G(E1,E2)}]$ will be significantly less than 1.0 and/or the genetic variances will not be equal between the groups ($\sigma_{gE1} \neq \sigma_{gE2}$) *(20,22)*.

To test for G×E interaction, a general model allowing for G×E interaction is compared, by use of maximum likelihood procedures, with a set of constrained (or restricted) models in which such interactions are excluded *(19,21)*. In the general model, environment 1 and environment 2 genetic standard deviations (σ_g), environment 1 and environment 2 environmental standard deviations (σ_e), and the genetic correlation between environment 1 and environment 2 (ρ_G) are estimated. The restricted models consist of a model in which the genetic correlation between environment 1 and environment 2 is constrained to 1.0 and a model in which the environment 1 and environment 2 genetic variances are constrained to be equal.

Each of the three restricted models is compared with the general model, to test whether the restricted model fits the data significantly worse than the general model using the likelihood ratio test. When comparing models with variances constrained to be equal, interpretation of significant differences are based on the assumption of an asymptotic χ_1^2 distribution for the likelihood test statistic. However, in the case of the model that restricted the genetic correlation to one, this assumption does not hold because the genetic correlation was constrained to the upper boundary of the parameter space ($\rho_G = 1.0$). As a result of this constraint, the test statistic is not distributed as an asymptotic χ_1^2, but rather as a one-half:one-half mixture of a χ_1^2 distribution and a point mass at zero *(5)*.

Three basic inferences concerning the nature of environment-based interactions can be made. The rejection of the model constraining the genetic correlation between the groups to equal one (i.e., $\rho_{G(E1,E2)}$ {not equal} 1.0) implies that a different gene or suite of genes is contributing to the variance in both environments. On the other hand, rejection of the model constraining the genetic standard deviations of the groups to be equal (i.e., $\sigma_{gE1} \neq \sigma_{gE2}$) would imply that the magnitude of the genetic effect is different in the two environments. It is the pattern of rejection or acceptance of these restricted models that gives insight into the precise mechanism of the interaction.

G×E tests are easily expanded to linkage analyses by simply modeling the genetic variance attributable to the QTL separately for each environment *(23)*. Therefore, the expected genetic covariance between a pair of relatives consisting of an individual from environment 1 and an individual from environment 2 is defined as

$$\text{COV}\left(G_{E1}, G_{E2}\right) = 2\phi \, \rho_{G(E1,E2)} \, \sigma_{gE1} \, \sigma_{gE2} + \Pi_q \sigma_{qE1} \, \sigma_{qE2}$$

where Π_q is a matrix whose elements (π_{qij}) provide the probability that individuals i and j are IBD at a QTL that is linked to a genetic marker locus and σ_{qE1} and σ_{qE2} are the marker-specific genetic standard deviations for environment 1 and 2, respectively. If there is a G×E interaction, then the marker-specific genetic standard deviations for environment 1 and 2 will be significantly different from each other. To assess G×E effects at a specific locus, this model will be compared with a linkage model in which the QTL variance is constrained to remain constant across environment. For each phenotype, the QTLs selected for analysis will be those identified in the initial univariate linkage analyses.

We performed an analysis looking at the interaction of environmental factors with a number of phenotypes in this cohort. In a first step, we tested within our German family dataset, including 1406 individuals in 514 families with MI, to determine whether there is an interaction between the environmental factor "smoking" on a number of cardiovascular risk factors (**Table 1**). For a detailed description of the phenotypes and the study populations, *see* Broeckel et al. *(24)*.

We detected a significant difference ($p > 0.05$) in the estimated genetic variation between smokers and nonsmokers for the phenotype diastolic blood pressure ($p > 0.05$). These findings suggest that in smokers compared with nonsmokers, different genes contribute to the phenotype. With regard to CAD, this analysis can easily be extended by analyzing the effect of risk factors on the phenotype of interest with regard to the influence of different or common shared genetic or environmental effects.

3. Conclusion

The described methods have been incorporated in the genetic analysis software package SOLAR, available at http://www.sfbr.org/solar/. Obviously, this chapter can give only a brief overview of the implemented analysis methods

Table 1
Gene–Environment Analysis for Smoking and Selected Cardiovascular Phenotypes

Trait	$\sigma_{G\,SMK}$	$\sigma_{G\,NSMK}$	$\sigma_{E\,SMK}$	$\sigma_{G\,NSMK}$	ρ_g	$\rho_g \neq 1$
Diastolic BP	3.61 ± 0.63	6.81 ± 1.62	7.04 ± 0.34	4.21 ± 2.24	−0.008 ± 0.49	$p < 0.05$
Heart rate	6.33 ± 0.89	5.35 ± 2.92	8.66 ± 0.58	9.84 ± 1.60	1.0	n.s.
Pulse pressure	7.15 ± 1.21	14.04 ± 2.95	12.94 ± 0.67	5.72 ± 6.02	0.60 ± 0.38	n.s.
Systolic BP	7.22 ± 1.59	13.56 ± 3.77	16.14 ± 0.76	10.97 ± 4.19	0.73 ± 0.55	n.s.

$\sigma_{G/E\,SMK}$ $\sigma_{G/E\,NSMK}$ denotes the genetic (g) and environmental (e) variance in smokers (SMK) vs nonsmokers (NSMK), respectively. BP, blood pressure.

available as part of this computer package. For a more detailed description of the analysis tools and additional features, we refer to the user manual and the listed references. It should be also noted that in order to extend the versatility of SOLAR software, tools have been developed to incorporate results from other programs, in particular IBD calculations using other estimation algorithms. Conversion programs are available to translate these files into SOLAR format.

Taken together, this SOLAR genetic analysis program package provides one of the most comprehensive analysis packages developed for statistical genetic analysis. Future development will focus on the analysis of SNP data in the context of family studies.

References

1. Merrill, R. M., Kessler, L. G., Udler, J. M., Rasband, G. C., and Feuer, E. J. (1999) Comparison of risk estimates for selected diseases and causes of death. *Prev. Med.* **28,** 179–193.
2. Colditz, G., Stampfer, M., Willett, W., Rosner, B., Speizer, F., and Hennekens, C. (1986) A prospective study of parental history of myocardial infarction and coronary heart disease in women. *Am. J. of Epidemiology* **123,** 48–58.
3. Schildkraut, J. M., Myers, R. H., Cupples, L. A., Kiely, D. K., and Kannel, W. B. (1989) Coronary risk associated with age and sex of parental heart disease in the Framingham Study. *Am. J. Cardiol.* **64,** 555–559.
4. Almasy, L. and Blangero, J. (1998) Multipoint quantitative-trait linkage analysis in general pedigrees. *Am. J. Hum. Genet.* **62,** 1198–1211.
5. Self, S. G. and Liang, K. Y. (1987) Asymptotic properties of maximum likelihood ratio tests under nonstandard conditions. *J. Am. Stat. Assc.* **82,** 605–610.
6. Schork, N. J. (1993) Extended multipoint identity-by-descent analysis of human quantitative traits: efficiency, power, and modeling considerations. *Am. J. Hum. Genet.* **53,** 1306–1319.
7. Williams, J. T., Duggirala, R., and Blangero, J. (1997) Statistical properties of a variance components method for quantitative trait linkage analysis in nuclear families and extended pedigrees. *Genet. Epidemiol.* **14,** 1065–1070.
8. Falkoner, D. S. (1989) *Introduction to Quantitative Genetics,* Longman Scientific and Technical, New York.
9. Sokal, R. R. and Rohlf, F. J. (1981) *Biometry: The Principles and Practice of Statistics in Biological Research,* WH Freeman and Company, San Francisco.
10. Almasy, L., Dyer, T. D., and Blangero, J. (1997) Bivariate quantitative trait linkage analysis: pleiotropy versus co-incident linkages. *Genet. Epidemiol.* **14,** 953–958.
11. Blangero, J., Williams, J. T., and Almasy, L. (2001) Variance component methods for detecting complex trait loci. *Adv. Genet.* **42,** 151–181.
12. Comuzzie, A. G., Mahaney, M., Almasy, L., Dyer, T. D., and Blangero, J. (1997) Exploiting pleiotropy to map genes for oligogenic phenotypes using extended pedigree data. *Genet. Epidemiol.* **14,** 975–980.

13. Mitchell, B. D., Ghosh, S., Schneider, J. L., Birznieks, G., and Blangero, J. (1997) Power of variance component linkage analysis to detect epistasis. *Genet. Epidemiol.* **14,** 1017–1022.

14. Amos, C. I. (1994) Robust variance-components approach for assessing genetic linkage in pedigrees. *Am. J. Hum. Genet.* **54,** 535–543.

15. Goldgar, D. (1990) Multipoint analysis of human quantitative genetic variation. *Am. J. Hum. Genet.* **47,** 957–967.

16. Amos, C. I., Zhu, D. K., and Boerwinkle, E. (1996) Assessing genetic linkage and association with robust components of variance approaches. *Ann. Hum. Genet.* **60,** 143–160.

17. Blangero, J. and Almasy, L. (1997) Multipoint oligogenic linkage analysis of quantitative traits. *Genet. Epidemiol.* **14,** 959–964.

18. Fulker, D. W., Cherny, S. S., and Cardon, L. R. (1995) Multipoint interval mapping of quantitative trait loci, using sib pairs. *Am. J. Hum. Genet.* **56,** 1224–1233.

19. Comuzzie, A. G., Blangero, J., Mahaney, M. C., Mitchell, B. D., Stern, M. P., and MacCluer, J. W. (1993) The quantitative genetics of sexual dimorphism in body fat measurements. *Am. J. Hum. Biol.* **5,** 725–734.

20. Robertson, A. (1959) The sampling variance of the genetic correlation coefficient. *Biometrics* **15,** 469-485.

21. Towne, B., Blangero, J., and Mott, G. E. (1992) Genetic analysis of sexual dimorphism in serum apo A1 and HDL-C concentrations in baboons. *Am. J. Primatol.* **27,** 107–117.

22. Eisen, E. and Legates, J. E. (1966) Genotype-sex interaction and the genetic correlation between the sexes for body weight in Mus musculus. *Genetics* **51,** 611–623.

23. Towne, B., Siervogel, R.M., and Blangero, J. (1997) Effects of genotype-by-sex interaction on quantitative trait linkage analysis. *Genet. Epidemiol.* **14,** 1053–1058.

24. Broeckel, U., Hengstenberg, C., Mayer, B., et al. (2002) A comprehensive linkage analysis for myocardial infarction and its related risk factors. *Nat. Genet.* **30,** 210–214.

8

Genome Resources and Comparative Analysis Tools for Cardiovascular Research

George E. Liu and Mark D. Adams

Summary

Disorders of the cardiovascular system are often caused by the interaction of genetic and environmental factors that jointly contribute to individual susceptibility. Genomic data and bioinformatics tools generated from genome projects, coupled with functional verification, offer novel approaches to study both rare single-gene and complex multigenic cardiovascular diseases. These approaches include gene mapping using genome variation, especially single-nucleotide polymorphisms and comparative genomics within and between species. This chapter illustrates the major genome resources, associated bioinformatics tools, and their potential application in cardiovascular research.

Key Words: Bioinformatics; genome browsers; genome applications; cardiovascular disease; comparative genomics; alignment algorithms.

1. Introduction

Although discovery of genes mutated in rare single-gene human diseases has become straightforward, it remains a hurdle to identify and determine the molecular mechanisms for complex multigenic human diseases such as myocardial infarction and congestive heart failure *(1)*. Those diseases are caused by the combined effects of multiple individual genes, none of which is responsible for the disease phenotype alone. The available complete human genome sequences *(2–4)* and bioinformatics tools offer us an unprecedented opportunity to study complex human diseases like cardiovascular (CV) diseases. Computational analysis and wet-bench verification experiments can be planned and conducted as two distinct but intertwined strategies. Large databases of genomic information, the interfaces to access them, and analytical methods for applying these data to particular biological problems have become increas-

From: *Methods in Molecular Medicine, Vol. 128: Cardiovascular Disease; Methods and Protocols; Volume 1*
Edited by: Q. Wang © Humana Press Inc., Totowa, NJ

ingly important tools to advance our understanding of CV development and pathogenesis and of interactions of genes with environment.

This chapter concentrates on the major genome resources and their associated comparative analysis tools. We will use the apolipoprotein A-V gene (*APOA5*) *(5)* and transcription factor gene *MEF2A (6)* as examples to illustrate their potential application in CV research.

2. Genomic Databases

The human genome sequence and associated information is available from three major public genomic browsers at the University of California at Santa Cruz (UCSC) *(7,8)*, the National Center for Biotechnology Information (NCBI) *(9–11)*, and Ensembl *(12–15)*. In each browser, the genome sequence is based on the same human genome assemblies prepared by NCBI (**Table 1**). Other species, including mouse, rat, and many others, are also incorporated in these genome browsers and updated regularly (*see* **Notes 1–3**). All three browsers provide a graphical user interface for accessing the genome sequences and navigating within the assemblies on the Internet. They provide keyword and sequence search tools to rapidly locate and retrieve the sequence data. Along the genomic sequence backbone, the browsers also provide other data known as "annotations." In addition to genes, the annotation includes chromosome banding, expressed sequence tags (ESTs), single-nucleotide polymorphisms (SNPs), and sequence-tagged sites (STSs), as well as comparative genomics and expression data. Each data item links out to other databases, websites, and published papers in PubMed. Sequences and annotations are downloadable in various formats for those wishing to do further analysis. With an emphasis on the application of gene mapping and comparative analysis in CV research, this section presents general guidelines for accessing the genome sequence and annotations using the three genome browsers.

2.1. UCSC Genome Browser

From the UCSC genome browser main page (http://genome.ucsc.edu/), users can search the genome in two basic ways: text searches and sequence similarity searches. The text search function in the Genome Browser Gateway allows searching by keywords such as gene name, gene symbol, ID, Genbank submitter name, chromosome number, chromosome region, proteins, clones, alleles, and bibliographic entries *(7,8)*. Sequence searches are performed using the alignment program BLAT *(16)*. Searches that identify a single result bring up the Genome Viewer page. Searches that retrieve multiple matches return an intermediary selection page listing all of the matched regions.

The Genome Viewer page of the human *APOA5* gene is organized in three portions: a Navigation section (**Fig. 1A**), a Data Display section (**Fig. 1B**), and

Table 1
Comparison of Three Major Genomic Browsers

Genome browser	UCSC	NCBI	Ensembl
Gene annotation			
Experimental evidence	SWISS-PROT, TrEMBL, and RefSeq	RefSeq, GenBan mRNAs, annotated known or potential transcripts, and EST sequences	SWISS-PROT, TrEMBL, and known protein, plus cDNA, and EST sequences
Gene prediction programs	Twinscan, SGP, GeneID, Genscan	Gnomon	Genewise, Genomewise, Genscan, Pmatch Supported by exp. evidence
Sequence mapping	BLAT, fast, less sensitive	BLAST, slow, more sensitive	BLAST, slow, more sensitive
Download interface	Table Browser	Perl scripts	EnsMart
Download format	Flat text, MySQL tables	Only flat text tables	FLAT TEXT, MySQL
Custom tracks	Custom tracks and DAS	No support	Custom tracks and DAS
Expression data	GNF, Affymetrix microarray data	SAGE data	GNF, Affymetrix microarray data, and EST-derived expression data

UCSC, University of California at Santa Cruz; NCBI, National Center for Biotechnology Information; EST, expressed sequence tag; DAS, Distributed Annotation Service; GNF, The Genomics Institute of the Novartis Research Foundation; GALA, Genome ALignments and Annotations.

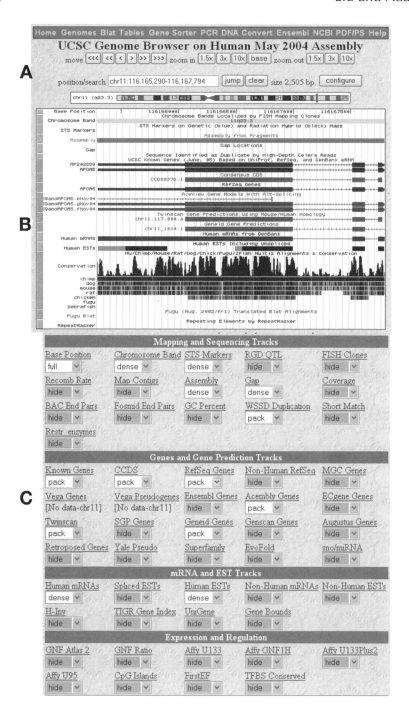

Fig. 1

a Feature Selection section (**Fig. 1C**). At the top (**Fig. 1A**) are (1) static links to the main searches, Home, FAQ, and Help pages; (2) general controls that zoom in or out, or slide right or left along the genome; and (3) the basic text search box. In the center (**Fig. 1B**) is the Data Display section of the genome viewer, which provides a dynamically generated graphical representation of the genome and the annotation as a stack of "tracks," each containing a type of annotation information or feature. The genome viewer displays information in related groups: **Mapping and Sequencing Tracks** (chromosome bands, assembly contigs and gaps, STSs), **Genes and Gene Prediction Tracks**, **mRNA and EST**, **Expression and Regulation**, **Comparative Genomics** (cross-species homologies), **ENCODE Tracks** *(17)*, and **Variation and Repeats** (SNPs and repetitive elements). At the bottom (**Fig. 1C**) there are grouped options to select features for individual annotation tracks in five modes: hide, dense, squish, pack, and full, which correspond to increasing levels of detail.

The Genome Viewer page can output selected regions of the genome (e.g., a gene) in GenBank, EMBL, XML, and other file formats. It allows selection of display options such as case, font, and color to represent annotations.

The UCSC genome browser also facilitates other search strategies. The Gene Sorter tool can be used to identify gene sets with similar characteristics such as sequence homology and expression pattern *(18)*. The PCR primer search returns the corresponding genomic sequence between two primers. The Table Browser is used to view sequence data and annotations in a text-based tabular format and to download them as tab-delimited flat files *(19)*.

2.2. NCBI Map Viewer

The NCBI Map Viewer (http://www.ncbi.nlm.nih.gov/mapview/) has been developed to represent gene information by position relative to other landmarks

---

Fig. 1. *(opposite page)* The Genome Viewer page of the human *APOA5* gene at the University of California at Santa Cruz genome browser. The display is organized in three sections: a Navigation section (**A**), a Data Display section (**B**), and a Feature Selection section (**C**). At the top (**A**) are the links to the main pages, general navigation controls within the genome, and the basic text search box. In the center (**B**) is the Data Display section of the genome viewer, which provides a graphical representation of the genome and the annotation as a stack of "tracks," each containing a type of annotation information or feature. The genome viewer displays information in related groups: Mapping and Sequencing, Genes and Gene Prediction, mRNA and Expressed Sequence Tag (EST), Expression and Regulation, Comparative Genomics, ENCODE, and Variation and Repeats Tracks. At the bottom (**C**) there are grouped options to select levels of detail for individual annotation tracks.

using map data. Currently, it contains genetic, radiation hybrid (RH), cyto-genetic, breakpoint, sequence-based, and clone maps for 29 organisms includ-ing human, mouse, and rat *(11)*. More importantly, the NCBI Map Viewer integrates these disparate maps by converting their inherent coordinate sys-tems into a single one based on the standard genome assembly. The correspon-dences between these maps in NCBI Map Viewer make it useful for identifying genes or gene families in a genomic region defined by genetic markers. Map Viewer also integrates seamlessly with other NCBI resources, like sequences in Entrez Gene, UniGene, Online Mendelian Inheritance in Man (OMIM), dbSNP, and dbSTS *(11,20–23)*. In a positional cloning project, when markers are placed on both genetic and sequence maps, it is then straight forward to use the gene-related maps (RefSeq, UniGene, ESTs, or *ab initio* gene predictions) *(11,24)* to identify possible genes of interest.

Figure 2 is a Map Viewer page of the human *APOA5* gene defined by a range of positions (chr11:116,135,000–116,215,000) as a query. On the top are Search and Find options (**Fig. 2A**). On the left of the page is an overview of the chromosome ideogram (**Fig. 2B**). The **Region Shown** and **Zoom** boxes con-trol the range displayed for the rightmost, or Master, Map in **Fig. 2D**. Explana-tion and tools are shown in **Fig. 2C**. **Maps & Options** links to a pop-up menu which allows one to fine-tune the region shown, the number and coordinate systems of maps, and the number of annotations on the Master Map, and to choose whether to show connections between maps. The **Fig. 2E** section pro-vides statistics of the elements mapped on the Master Map.

The maps are displayed vertically in **Fig. 2D**. Features displayed on the Master Map (rightmost) have brief descriptive labels; information on features on the non-Master Maps can be found by placing the mouse over an object. The labels on the Master Map depend on the type of object and maps being explored, but generally provide: (1) links to resources defining the mapped element, e.g., Entrez Gene records; (2) the direction of transcription for genes; (3) the evidence or confidence in the placement or sequence in the region; and (4) links to view the Online Mendelian Inheritance in Man (**OMIM**) records, to view the DNA sequence (sequence viewer [**sv**]), to view the protein sequences (protein [**pr**]), to download the sequence (download [**dl**]), to view the EST/mRNA alignments in a region (evidence viewer [**ev**]), to view homol-ogy maps (HomoloGene [**hm**]) *(11)*, and to create cDNA sequences in real time (Model Maker [**mm**]). The Map Viewer can generate a Table View of the current display for export to other programs. Segments of a genomic assembly may be downloaded using the Map Viewer's "Download/View Sequence/Evi-dence" link in either GenBank or FASTA formats.

Using the ortholog gene relations provided through NCBI's HomoloGene, the Map Viewer can also align maps from more than one organism to facilitate comparative analysis.

2.3. Ensembl

Ensembl (http://www.ensembl.org/) is an open-source project for developing a portable system to handle data storage, analysis, and visualization of large genomes. It has the most sophisticated gene prediction pipelines and, as a result, the Ensembl viewers and annotations are gene-oriented. The Ensembl project can easily facilitate a gene-centric study such as mapping a candidate gene or gene families to a specific region and identifying the genes and SNPs within the region. The EnsMart interface also allows more complex questions to be asked to identify genes with a user-defined set of characteristics.

Ensembl provides access to its genome data and annotations in three ways: (1) the Ensembl website by keywords or sequence similarity searches; (2) a web-based data-mining interface called EnsMart; and (3) *en masse* downloadable datasets or direct access to its MySQL databases.

The Ensembl website provides a variety of views of the genome data. A **ContigView** of the human Chr11q23.3 region containing the *APOA5* gene is shown in **Fig. 3**. At the top are the general links and search box (**Fig. 3A**) and **Chromosome** panel showing the region of interest in chromosome 11 (**Fig. 3B**). In the middle, the **Overview** panel shows the 1 Mb region of interest with overlaid markers and genes (**Fig. 3C**). The lower **Detailed View** panel shows 80 kb of genomic sequence features in detail (chr11:116,135,000–116,215,000, **Fig. 3D**), including five types of transcripts. There is redundancy among these predictions and they are listed in deceasing order of preference/quality: (1) known transcripts; (2) Vega transcripts from the Vertebrate Genome Annotation (VEGA) database *(25)*; (3) Ensembl transcripts predicted using at least one experimental evidence by Ensembl; (4) EST transcripts predicted using only EST evidence by Ensembl; and (5) GENSCAN transcripts predicted by an *ab initio* computer program. The genome is central in the panel, with the forward strand on the top and the reverse on the bottom. Like the UCSC genome browser, there are control bars for navigation and zooming within the genomes. The pull-down menus allow the user to hide and display the detailed features. They also allow the addition of comparative tracks and annotation from third-party sources.

The Ensembl website supplies other view pages, including: **MapView**, displaying the chromosome ideogram along with feature density plots for genes, GC content, repetitive sequences, and SNPs; **GeneView**, showing individual

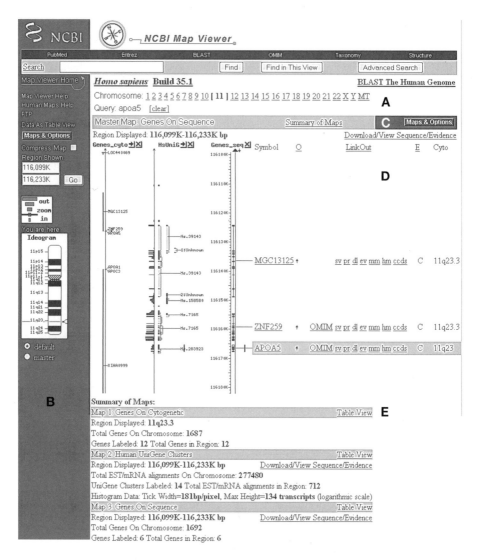

Fig. 2. The Map Viewer page of the human *APOA5* gene at the National Center for Biotechnology Information. A range of sequence coordinates (chr11:116,135,000–116,215,000) was used as a query. On the top are Search and Find options (**A**). On the left of the page is an overview of the chromosome ideogram (**B**). The Region Shown and Zoom boxes control the range displayed for the rightmost, or Master, Map in **D**. Explanation and tools are shown in **C**. Maps & Options links to a pop-up menu which fine-tunes the region shown, the number and coordinate systems of maps, whether to show connections between maps, and the number of annotations on the Master Map. The **E** section provides statistics of the elements mapped on the Master Map.

Ensembl genes with transcripts and gene structures; and **ProteinView**, showing individual Ensembl translations with functional annotation from InterPro. Recent additions to Ensembl are **SyntenyView**, **MultiContigView**, and **GeneSNPView**. The **SyntenyView** shows conservation of large-scale gene order between two or more genomes. The **MultiContigView** page displays aligned regions of genomes from multiple species. It is able to display both DNA similarity and putative ortholog gene relationships. The **GeneSNPView** web page centralizes all information of genome variations (SNPs) for a single gene from DNA, RNA, and protein levels into one page *(15)*.

To facilitate rapid retrieval of customized data sets from large genomes, **EnsMart** (http://www.ensembl.org/Multi/martview) was developed to allow easy data mining via the **MartView** web interface *(26)*. The system consists of a query-optimized database and interactive, user-friendly interfaces supporting complex queries on various types of annotations for numerous species. For more details, *see* **Subheading 2.6.** Results of tabulated data or biological sequence can be output dynamically, in HTML, text, Microsoft Excel, and compressed formats.

2.4. Genome Browser Features and Comparisons

A simple comparison of the three major genomic browsers is presented in **Table 1** to provide a starting point for users.

2.4.1. Gene Prediction

The three genomic browsers have different annotation of genes on the assembled sequences. For example, for the location or numbers of both known and predicted genes, different browsers may use different sources of mRNA for their known genes, different methods to localize the mRNAs in the genome, different gene prediction tools, and different means of reaching a consensus gene structure. Although the algorithms are being continuously refined, the quality of prediction is restricted by both the software and the available experimental data. Therefore, it is always important to rely on experimental evidence to make a sound decision about the accuracy of putative genes, especially ones predicted *ab initio*.

The Comparative Genomics tracks also may help to define functional regions under evolutionary constraints (*see* **Subheading 3.5.**). The UCSC genome browser separates the gene annotations based on the type of evidence. In the NCBI Map Viewer, the Genes_Sequence track shows all gene models, both with and without mRNA evidence. The *ab initio* transcript and EST maps, as well as the model maker or evidence viewer are designed to help users in their evaluations. Ensembl predictions can be evaluated in the GeneView and TransView for individual genes and transcripts, as well as by adding additional

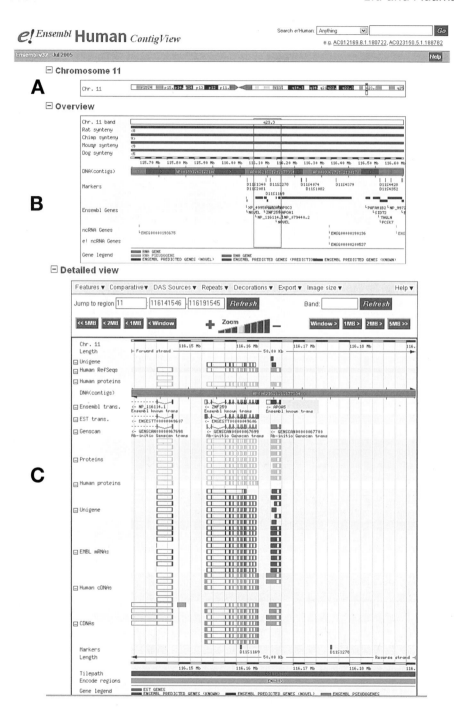

Fig. 3.

transcript and protein features to the ContigView. Each browser presents only one view of a given genome. In many cases, it may be useful to look at and compare the same region of the genome in more than one browser.

2.4.2. Interfaces and Speed

Users may find that different browsers are better for different queries. Sequence-based queries often runs faster in the UCSC Genome Browser than in the others. UCSC uses the less sensitive but much faster BLAT program *(16)*, whereas both NCBI and Ensembl use BLAST *(27)* to perform sequence searches.

2.4.3. Custom Tracks

Both UCSC and Ensembl allow users to display their own data, and support Distributed Annotation Service (DAS) protocol *(28)* to allow users to share their data with others; NCBI Map Viewer does not support this. However, NCBI provides more nonsequence-based maps.

2.4.4. Expression Data

The UCSC Browser and Ensembl provide links to the microarray expression data generated by the Genomics Institute of the Novartis Foundation at http://expression.gnf.org/cgi-bin/index.cgi *(29,30)*, whereas NCBI MapViewer does not. In contrast, NCBI's MapViewer displays SAGE tag information instead *(31)*.

2.4.5. Download

All of the data presented in the genome browsers are also available for download from the respective sites. At present, UCSC provides flat text files, as well as MySQL tables. NCBI provides only text files. Ensembl provides flat text files, as well as database tables ready for loading into MySQL. Furthermore,

---

Fig. 3. *(opposite page)* A ContigView page of the human Chr11q23.3 region containing the *APOA5* gene at Ensembl. At the top are the general links and search box (**A**) and Chromosome panel showing the region of interest in chromosome 11 (**B**). In the middle, the Overview panel shows the 1-Mb region of interest with overlaid markers and genes (**C**). The lower Detailed View panel shows 80 kb (chr11:116,135,000-116,215,000) of genomic sequence features in details (**D**), including five types of transcripts. The genome, is central in the panel, with the forward strand on the top and the reverse on the bottom. Control bars allow navigation and zooming within the genomes. The pull-down menus allow the user to hide and display the detailed features. They also allow the addition of comparative tracks and annotation from third party sources.

all Ensembl software, including the code used to generate the website, is freely available.

2.5. Example 1

As a CV gene mapping example, Wang et al. *(6)* performed a genome-wide linkage scan with 382 markers and identified chromosome 15q26 as a coronary artery disease (CAD) and myocardial infarction (MI) locus. Further haplotype analysis with neighboring markers verified the observed linkage. Known and putative genes located in the locus (*see* **ref. 6** and Fig. 1 and Table S2 therein) were compiled by searching the UCSC Genome Browser, the GeneMap99 Database and UniGene Database at NCBI. Based on biological evidence and the Mendelian, autosomal-dominant inheritance model, the candidate gene *MEF2A* was chosen to screen for mutations using direct DNA sequence analysis. Based on their results, the authors concluded that the deletion of 21 bp in transcription factor gene *MEF2A* causes an autosomal dominant form of CAD/ MI. Since then, another independent group identified new *MEF2A* mutations in a CAD population *(32)*. There was also a study reporting a contradictory result *(18)*. The discrepancy could be due to different case–control classification, reduced penetrance, and the effects of a genetic or environmental modifier. These conflicting results illustrate the difficulty of connecting genetic variation to common diseases *(33)*.

2.6. Example 2

Candidate gene identification is a labor-intensive task in the dissection of complex genetic diseases. First, researchers narrow down the disease gene to a region of the genome by comparing individuals with the disease with matched unaffected controls using a combination of genotyping and statistical approaches. The region is then subjected to a detailed examination to identify candidate genes in the disease phenotype. Because researchers already know in which tissues the causative gene is expected to be expressed and what its potential function may be, EnsMart can greatly facilitate this process by applying genomic region, expression pattern, and protein function filters and prioritize the potential genes to be screened.

SNP selection is another tedious task, requiring data retrieval, filtering, and selection from raw resources such as dbSNP *(23,34,35)*. EnsMart allows quick identification of suitable SNPs (for example, with a reasonable minor allele frequency in the study population) to screen for a gene association with the disease. The dbSNP database can be queried by EnsMart on SNP IDs and attributes such as their validation status; their location in the coding, intronic, or upstream conserved noncoding regions; and whether they are synonymous or nonsynonymous if located in protein-coding regions.

3. Programs for Genomic Applications and Comparative Genomics Resources

The National Heart, Lung, and Blood Institute (NHLBI) initiated the Programs for Genomic Applications (PGAs; http://www.nhlbi.nih.gov/resources/pga/index.htm) in September 2000 as a major initiative to advance functional genomics related to heart, lung, blood, and sleep health and disorders. These PGAs develop information, tools, and resources to link genes to biological function on a genomic scale and share all the information, reagents, and tools freely and quickly. Several PGAs are related to CV health and disorders. These PGAs explore broad and multidisciplinary approaches to understanding genetic characteristics of normal and abnormal CV functions.

3.1. Berkeley PGA

The Berkeley PGA, led by Dr. Eddy Rubin at The Lawrence Berkeley National Laboratory (http://pga.lbl.gov/) and entitled **Comparative Genomic Analysis of Cardiovascular Gene Regulation**, is particularly interesting for CV researchers. In multigenic CV diseases, one important aspect is the temporal, spatial, or quantitative changes in the expression of individual genes. Instead of concentrating on gene discovery, this PGA focuses on identifying and functionally characterizing regulatory regions in the expression of CV related genes. It is expected that comparative genomics will function as the most direct, global, and cost-effective approach to identifying transcriptional regulatory elements embedded in genomic sequence. This PGA is aiming to analyze 200 human and 200 mouse orthologous genomic intervals. They developed the VISTA Genome Browser (http://pipeline.lbl.gov/) to perform sequence alignment, analysis, and interactive visualization of conservation between large genomes with multiple annotation and display options *(36,37)*. The VISTA tracks can also be overlaid onto the UCSC genome browser to facilitate a comparison of conservation features using different algorithms in the context of the many other whole genome annotations not present on the VISTA genome browser such as transcription factor binding sites.

The resultant sequence alignments and annotations around CV-related genes are publicly available from Cardiovascular Comparative Genomic Database (CVCGD; http://pga.lbl.gov/cvcgd.html). The database contains information like Gene name, Gene ID in the OMIM database (**OMIM**), Human map location (**HM**), GenBank accession number for human cDNA (**HC**), Mouse map location (**MM**), and GenBank accession number for mouse cDNA (**MC**). Users can search CVCGD by gene name and abbreviation, alphabetically or by categories (groups of diseases). This database can function as a start point to design and perform functional verification of hypotheses derived from the comparative analysis.

3.2. Example 3

As a side product of an effort to scan evolutionarily conserved sequences in the well-characterized *APOA1/C3/A4* gene cluster on human 11q23, researchers from the Berkeley PGA detected a genomic interval with extended interspecies sequence conservation *(5)*. Its VISTA graphical plot displays the level of homology between human and the orthologous mouse sequence (*see* **ref. 5**, Fig. 1 therein). Based on the results from EST sampling and Northern blots, they identified a novel apolipoprotein-like gene (*APOA5*), which is used as an example in this chapter. They further verified the function of *APOA5* using transgenic mice (both with *APOA5* gene knock-in and knockout) and genetic association studies between human *APOAV* polymorphisms and lipid level.

3.3. Related PGAs

Other interesting PGAs include **Mouse Models of Heart, Lung, and Blood Diseases** in Jackson Laboratory (JAX PGA at http://pga.jax.org/), **The Bay Area Functional Genomics Consortium** at the University of California at San Francisco (BayGenomics PGA at http://baygenomics.ucsf.edu/) and **Physiogenomics of Stressors in Derived Consomic Rats & Knock-Out Rats for Physiological Genomics** in Medical College of Wisconsin (PhysGen PGA at http://pga.mcw.edu/). Using large-scale phenotype driven single nucleotide mutagenesis screens of mice *(38)*, the JAX PGA is aiming to identify genes and interacting gene networks that underlie several diseases including hypertension. As a complement to the above approach, the BayGenomics PGA and other members of the International Gene Trap Consortium (http://www.genetrap.org) are using custom gene-trap vectors as a source of insertional mutagenesis with an eventual goal of providing a knockout resource for each mouse gene *(39)*. The PhysGen PGA (http://pga.mcw.edu/) is focused on understanding the genetic basis of fundamental mechanistic pathways of the heart, lung, kidney, blood and vasculature through development of consomic rat panels and knockout models and physiological genomics, using environmental stressors. Interested readers should refer to their websites for more information.

3.4. Rodent Genome Databases

Mice and rats are well suited to the study of complex genetic diseases. The following databases contain considerable information on rodent models of CV disease. The Mouse Genome Informatics (MGI) system at The Jackson Laboratory (http://www.informatics.jax.org) provides integrated access to data on the genetics, genomics, and biology of the laboratory mouse *(40–42)*. One core component of MGI is Mouse Genome Database (MGD), which contains mouse genes, genetic markers, and genomic features as well as their associations with sequence sets, reagents, alleles, and mutant strains. It also includes comparative and experimental mapping data, and integration of cytogenetic, linkage, and physical maps. MGI also includes the Mouse Phenome Database (MPD) *(43,44)*. Reliable and consistent phenotypic data, which are ready to compare in a cost-effective way, are essential for the full utility of genotypic information from genome projects. The MPD project promotes the quantitative phenotypic characterization of commonly used and genetically diverse inbred mouse strains under standardized conditions. Forty inbred strains and wild-derived inbred strains were carefully chosen for initial testing, and MPD was developed to store, access, and analyze these phenotypic data. Haplotype maps of inbred mouse strains accompanied by delineation of their phenotypic variation and gene expression patterns will definitely speed up complex trait analysis. As of May 2005, MGI contains 932 alleles, 695 genes/markers, and 97 quantitative trait loci (QTLs), which are related to CV system phenotype. Similarly to MGD, the Rat Genome Database (RGD) at Medical College of Wisconsin (http://rgd.mcw.edu) collects and consolidates rat genetic, genomic, and biological resources including rat genes, QTLs, microsatellite markers, and rat strains. RGD also integrates with the rat genomic sequence to provide a disease-centric resource, applicable to human and mouse via comparative analysis. As of May 2005, RGD contains approx 300 CV-related rat QTLs. The current development of RGD is toward creating a rat phenome database.

3.5. Comparative Genomics Algorithms

Different algorithms, such as BLASTZ, MULTIZ, LAGAN, Multi-LAGAN, Shuffle-LAGAN, AVID, and TBA *(45–49)* have been used to generate genomic alignments on selected organisms, and these precomputed alignments can be viewed in the UCSC, Ensembl, and VISTA genome browsers. The browsers display histograms indicating the conservation score, calculated using various models within pairwise or multiple alignments of orthologous genome regions.

The UCSC and Ensembl genome browsers use BLASTZ, MULTIZ, and phastCons. BLASTZ extends initial matching seeds using a gradually decreased threshold system to extend the contiguity of the final alignments *(45)*. Best-in-genome pairwise alignments were generated for each species using BLASTZ and ordered along the chromosomes. The pairwise alignments were then multiply aligned using MULTIZ. The resulting multiple alignments were then assigned conservation scores by phastCons based on a Phylogenetic hidden Markov models (phylo-HMM) *(50–52)*.

In the VISTA genome browser, pairwise or multiple alignments can be prepared by LAGAN, Multi-LAGAN, Shuffle-LAGAN, or AVID *(46–48)*. LAGAN first determines the best local alignments as anchors to limit the search space and then focuses on aligning and finally connecting the regions between the anchors to prepare the global alignments. As a result, the speed of LAGAN is improved dramatically compared to other algorithms. Based on LAGAN, Multi-LAGAN generates multiple genomic sequence alignments, such as ClustalW, using a progressive alignment approach guided by a phylogenetic tree *(46)* (*see* **Note 4**). The AVID program *(48)* also is a global approach that is able to detect weak homologies. Its other features include large capacity, accuracy, and ability to handle the draft sequences (by ordering and orienting the contigs automatically). Like LAGAN, AVID relies on the use of strong anchors. After the initial set of anchors is identified, the regions between the anchors are realigned and new anchors are selected. The process continues recursively until all sequences are aligned, making the speed of AVID relatively slower.

3.6. Servers for Large-Scale Genomic Alignments

Users can generate custom large-scale genomic alignments using the following web severs or associated tools.

3.6.1. PipMaker

PipMaker (http://pipmaker.bx.psu.edu/pipmaker/) uses the BLASTZ Program to align two very long genomic DNA sequences with one another, and is available through both a Web front-end and a downloadable executable *(53,54)*. After being submitted, the PipMaker server will return a percent identity plot (pip) in PDF or PostScript format, as well as any text-based alignments using E-mail. The PipMaker server does not have a maximum length limit on the sequences submitted, but does tend to time out for sequences longer than 2 Mbp. The input to PipMaker consists of two sequences in FASTA format, along with optional annotation files for repeats and exons. The genomic sequences can be aligned in the forward direction, or the first sequence can be aligned with both directions of the second sequence.

3.6.2. VISTA

The VISTA server (http://genome.lbl.gov/vista/index.shtml) allows two or more genomic sequences of interest to be aligned using an algorithm chosen from AVID, LAGAN, or Shuffle-LAGAN *(46,47)*. Unlike PipMaker, VISTA detects repetitive sequences and does not depend on the repeats file supplied by users. VISTA produces smooth graphs to represent the conservation level using a sliding window scheme. The sliding window length can be customized to calculate percent identities (default of 100 bp) and so can the minimum conservation level to show on the plot (default 50%). The sequences are aligned in both the forward and reversed directions, as specified in the FASTA input files.

Several versions of VISTA exist *(37,55)*: rVISTA can identify potential transcription factor binding sites *(56,57)*; cVISTA runs the normal VISTA in complement mode to study sequence differences between species (i.e., Phylogenetic shadowing) *(58,59)*; GenomeVISTA allows a query sequence to be mapped on the precomputed whole-genome assemblies; PhyloVISTA provides an interactive interface for analyzing multiple phylogenetic frameworks.

3.6.3. zPicture and Mulan

As a second generation of comparative sequence analysis and visualization tools, zPicture runs significantly faster than PipMaker and VISTA *(49)*. Instead of using E-mail to reply, zPicture (http://zpicture.dcode.org/) provides a dynamic Web-based interface to analyze the conservation profiles by allowing the critical parameters to be adjusted interactively. It is able to automatically fetch and format sequences and gene annotations from the UCSC genome browser. It also interacts with rVista (http://rvista.dcode.org) to facilitate transcription factor binding-site analysis. zPicture utilizes the BLASTZ program to perform pairwise alignments. Alignments can be visualized either in standard pip (percent identity plot) or in Vista-style graphs. Similarly, Mulan (http://mulan.dcode.org/) is a local sequence alignment and visualization tool for multiple sequence alignments based on the TBA algorithm *(49,60)*.

3.7. Additional Resources

3.7.1. Other Chapters of Interest

This chapter concentrates on the major genome resources and their associated analysis tools in the context of CV gene mapping analysis and comparative genomics. For other relevant topics, readers should refer to the other chapters in this book. For additional methodological details on approaches to gene mapping, please refer to Chapter 2. The genotyping markers can be retrieved from NCBI's dbSNP (http://www.ncbi.nlm.nih.gov/SNP) *(35)* and the HapMap project (http://www.hapmap.org/) *(61)*. Biolgoical annotation in the form of assessing the location, timing, and dependencies of gene expression is a major area of functional genomics and we refer readers to Chapter 4. Two relevant databases for genome-wide expression profiling can be found at The Genomics Institute of the Novartis Research Foundation (GNF) (http://expression.gnf.org/cgi-bin/index.cgi) and the Gene Expression Omnibus (http://www.ncbi.nlm.nih.gov/geo/).

3.7.2. Additional Databases

There are additional resources which we do not cover, such as the Genome ALignments and Annotations (GALA) database *(62,63)*, the GO project *(64–*

68), and the STRING database *(69,70)*. GALA is a relational database to contain information on genomic sequence similarities as well as functional elements in DNA and experimental results that demonstrate those functions. Currently, it includes five vertebrate species: human, chimpanzee, mouse, rat, and chicken. It supports simple and complex queries, such as clustering and searching elements, as well as set subtraction and intersections. The database is available online at http://www.bx.psu.edu/. The goal of the Gene Ontology project (http://www.geneontology.org/) is to produce a controlled vocabulary that facilitates the communication among the research community. It provides three structured networks of defined terms to describe gene product attributes. They are **molecular function, biological process**, and **cellular component**. It is widely used and facilitates comparison of gene information among annotated genomes. At the protein level, direct (physical) and indirect (functional) associations of gene products/proteins can be retrieved from the Search Tool for the Retrieval of Interacting Genes/Proteins (STRING) at http://string. embl.de/.

3.7.3. Websites

Genome databases and browsers:
http://genome.ucsc.edu/cgi-bin/hgGateway; UCSC Genome Browser
http://www.ncbi.nlm.nih.gov/mapview/; NCBI Map Viewer
http://www.ensembl.org/; ENSEMBL
http://www.ensembl.org/Multi/martview; Ensembl EnsMart Genome Browser
     (MartView)
http://pipeline.lbl.gov/cgi-bin/gateway2; VISTA Genome Browser

Comparative genomics and tools:
http://www.bx.psu.edu/miller_lab/; BLASTZ, MULTIZ and TBA alignment programs
http://pipmaker.bx.psu.edu/pipmaker/; PipMaker and MultiPipMaker
http://lagan.stanford.edu/lagan_web/index.shtml; LAGAN/Multi-LAGAN
http://genome.lbl.gov/vista/index.shtml; VISTA/AVID
http://zpicture.dcode.org; zPicture
http://mulan.dcode.org; Mulan
http://rvista.dcode.org; rVISTA

Programs for genomic applications:
http://www.nhlbi.nih.gov/resources/pga/index.htm; NHLBI's PGA website
http://pga.lbl.gov/; Berkeley PGA at LBNL
http://pga.lbl.gov/cvcgd.html; Berkeley PGA's CVCGD
http://pga.jax.org/; JAX PGA at Jackson Laboratory
http://pga.mcw.edu/; PhysGen PGA at Medical College of Wisconsin
http://baygenomics.ucsf.edu/; BayGenomics PGA at UCSF

SNP and HapMap:

http://www.ncbi.nlm.nih.gov/SNP; dbSNP
http://www.hapmap.org/; the HapMap project

Gene expression databases:
http://expression.gnf.org/cgi-bin/index.cgi; The Genomics Institute of the Novartis
    Research Foundation (GNF) database
http://www.ncbi.nlm.nih.gov/geo/; Gene Expression Omnibus

Additional resources:
    http://www.bx.psu.edu/; GALA database
    http://www.geneontology.org/; the GO (Gene Ontology) project
    http://string.embl.de/; STRING database

4. Notes

1. The genome assemblies that form the basis of the genome browsers are dynamic
   in nature, and updates occur occasionally for human and more frequently for
   mouse, rat, and other organisms. Therefore, when making comparisons among
   browsers, it is important to check that the same assembly of the genome is being
   used. Changes in sequence data (additions that fill gaps and change the order of
   genome segments) or algorithmic improvements can sometimes cause large
   changes in the assembly. From assembly to assembly, genes can move within or
   between chromosomes; genomic coordinates may change along the chromosome;
   new fragments can shift from unknown portions into the assembly. In extreme
   cases, the assembly may not be correct, especially for telomere and centromere
   regions, because of limitations of the assembly algorithm or errors in the underlying data. These cases may require further investigation and even focused
   resequencing.
2. The UCSC browser is currently the only one of the three sites to provide a graphical interface to older versions of the assembly. Its frequently updated Help and
   News pages describe features, changes, and the current state of the genome
   sequence assemblies. Ensembl provides a "preview" browser for organisms
   whose genomes are in early stages of assembly and annotation.
3. Each assembly version is identified by its build number or by a date; for example,
   the human genome assembly completed in May 2004 is referred to as "NCBI
   Build 35" and as "hg17" at UCSC. When referring to a particular genome region
   by its coordinates on a chromosome, it is essential to know which assembly version is being referenced.
4. The complete Ensembl software system for manipulating and storing genome
   information is freely available with source code for others to use.
5. Compared with ClustalW, Multi-LAGAN runs much faster. Shuffle-LAGAN is
   a modified version of LAGAN that is able to find rearrangements (inversions,
   transpositions, and some duplications) in a global alignment framework *(47)*. It
   uses CHAOS *(71)* local alignments to build a map of the rearrangements between
   the sequences, and LAGAN to align the regions of conserved synteny.

References

1. Botstein, D. and Risch, N. (2003) Discovering genotypes underlying human phenotypes: past successes for mendelian disease, future approaches for complex disease. *Nat. Genet.* **33(Suppl)**, 228–237.
2. Lander, E. S., Linton, L. M., Birren, B., et al. (2001) Initial sequencing and analysis of the human genome. *Nature* **409**, 860–921.
3. Venter, J. C., Adams, M. D., Myers, E. W., et al. (2001) The sequence of the human genome. *Science* **291**, 1304–1351.
4. The International Human Genome Sequencing Consortium. (2004) Finishing the euchromatic sequence of the human genome. *Nature* **431**, 931–945.
5. Pennacchio, L. A., Olivier, M., Hubacek, J. A., et al. (2001) An apolipoprotein influencing triglycerides in humans and mice revealed by comparative sequencing. *Science* **294**, 169–173.
6. Wang, L., Fan, C., Topol, S. E., Topol, E. J., and Wang, Q. (2003) Mutation of MEF2A in an inherited disorder with features of coronary artery disease. *Science* **302**, 1578–1581.
7. Karolchik, D., Baertsch, R., Diekhans, M., et al. (2003) The UCSC Genome Browser Database. *Nucleic Acids Res.* **31**, 51–54.
8. Kent, W. J., Sugnet, C. W., Furey, T. S., et al. (2002) The human genome browser at UCSC. *Genome Res.* **12**, 996–1006.
9. Wheeler, D. L., Church, D. M., Federhen, S., et al. (2003) Database resources of the National Center for Biotechnology. *Nucleic Acids Res.* **31**, 28–33.
10. Wheeler, D. L., Church, D. M., Edgar, R., et al. (2004) Database resources of the National Center for Biotechnology Information: update. *Nucleic Acids Res.* **32**, D35–D40.
11. Wheeler, D. L., Barrett, T., Benson, D. A., et al. (2005) Database resources of the National Center for Biotechnology Information. *Nucleic Acids Res.* **33**, D39–D45.
12. Hubbard, T., Barker, D., Birney, E., et al. (2002) The Ensembl genome database project. *Nucleic Acids Res.* **30**, 38–41.
13. Clamp, M., Andrews, D., Barker, D., et al. (2003) Ensembl 2002: accommodating comparative genomics. *Nucleic Acids Res.* **31**, 38–42.
14. Birney, E., Andrews, D., Bevan, P., et al. (2004) Ensembl 2004. *Nucleic Acids Res.* **32**, D468–D470.
15. Hubbard, T., Andrews, D., Caccamo, M., et al. (2005) Ensembl 2005. *Nucleic Acids Res.* **33**, D447–D453.
16. Kent, W. J. (2002) BLAT—the BLAST-like alignment tool. *Genome Res.* **12**, 656-664.
17. ENCODE Project Consortium. (2004) The ENCODE (ENCyclopedia Of DNA Elements) Project. *Science* **306**, 636–640.
18. Weng, L., Kavaslar, N., Ustaszewska, A., et al. (2005) Lack of MEF2A mutations in coronary artery disease. *J. Clin. Invest.* **115**, 1016–1020.
19. Karolchik, D., Hinrichs, A. S., Furey, T. S., et al. (2004) The UCSC Table Browser data retrieval tool. *Nucleic Acids Res.* **32**, D493–D496.

20. Hamosh, A., Scott, A. F., Amberger, J. S., Bocchini, C. A., and McKusick, V. A. (2005) Online Mendelian Inheritance in Man (OMIM), a knowledgebase of human genes and genetic disorders. *Nucleic Acids Res.* **33,** D514–D517.
21. Thorisson, G. A. and Stein, L. D. (2003) The SNP Consortium website: past, present and future. *Nucleic Acids Res.* **31,** 124–127.
22. Maglott, D., Ostell, J., Pruitt, K. D., and Tatusova, T. (2005) Entrez Gene: gene-centered information at NCBI. *Nucleic Acids Res.* **33,** D54–D58.
23. Smigielski, E. M., Sirotkin, K., Ward, M., and Sherry, S. T. (2000) dbSNP: a database of single nucleotide polymorphisms. *Nucleic Acids Res.* **28,** 352–355.
24. Pruitt, K. D., Tatusova, T., and Maglott, D. R. (2005) NCBI Reference Sequence (RefSeq): a curated non-redundant sequence database of genomes, transcripts and proteins. *Nucleic Acids Res.* **33,** D501–D504.
25. Ashurst, J. L., Chen, C. K., Gilbert, J. G., et al. (2005) The Vertebrate Genome Annotation (Vega) database. *Nucleic Acids Res.* **33,** D459–D465.
26. Kasprzyk, A., Keefe, D., Smedley, D., et al. (2004) EnsMart: a generic system for fast and flexible access to biological data. *Genome Res.* **14,** 160–169.
27. Altschul, S. F., Gish, W., Miller, W., Myers, E. W., and Lipman,D.J. (1990) Basic local alignment search tool. *J. Mol. Biol.* **215,** 403–410.
28. Dowell, R. D., Jokerst, R. M., Day, A., Eddy, S. R., and Stein, L. (2001) The distributed annotation system. *BMC Bioinformatics.* **2,** 7.
29. Su, A. I., Cooke, M. P., Ching, K. A., et al. (2002) Large-scale analysis of the human and mouse transcriptomes. *Proc. Natl. Acad. Sci. USA* **99,** 4465–4470.
30. Su, A. I., Wiltshire, T., Batalov, S., et al. (2004) A gene atlas of the mouse and human protein-encoding transcriptomes. *Proc. Natl. Acad. Sci. USA* **101,** 6062–6067.
31. Velculescu, V. E., Zhang, L., Vogelstein, B., and Kinzler, K. W. (1995) Serial analysis of gene expression. *Science* **270,** 484–487.
32. Gonzalez, P., Garcia-Castro, M., Reguero, J. R., et al. (2006) The Pro279Leu variant in the transcription factor MEF2A is associated with myocardial infarction. *J. Med. Genet.* **43(2),** 167–169.
33. Altshuler, D. and Hirschhorn, J. N. (2005) MEF2A sequence variants and coronary artery disease: a change of heart? *J. Clin. Invest.* **115,** 831–833.
34. Sherry, S. T., Ward, M., and Sirotkin, K. (2000) Use of molecular variation in the NCBI dbSNP database. *Hum. Mutat.* **15,** 68–75.
35. Sherry, S. T., Ward, M. H., Kholodov, M., et al. (2001) dbSNP: the NCBI database of genetic variation. *Nucleic Acids Res.* **29,** 308–311.
36. Mayor, C., Brudno, M., Schwartz, J. R., et al. (2000) VISTA: visualizing global DNA sequence alignments of arbitrary length. *Bioinformatics* **16,** 1046–1047.
37. Frazer, K. A., Pachter, L., Poliakov, A., Rubin, E. M., and Dubchak, I. (2004) VISTA: computational tools for comparative genomics. *Nucleic Acids Res.* **32,** W273–W279.
38. Nadeau, J. H. and Frankel, W. N. (2000) The roads from phenotypic variation to gene discovery: mutagenesis versus QTLs. *Nat. Genet.* **25,** 381–384.

39. Skarnes, W. C., von Melchner, H., Wurst, W., et al. (2004) A public gene trap resource for mouse functional genomics. *Nat. Genet.* **36,** 543–544.

40. Blake, J. A., Richardson, J. E., Bult, C. J., Kadin, J. A., and Eppig, J. T. (2002) The Mouse Genome Database (MGD): the model organism database for the laboratory mouse. *Nucleic Acids Res.* **30,** 113–115.

41. Bult, C. J., Blake, J. A., Richardson, J. E., et al. (2004) The Mouse Genome Database (MGD): integrating biology with the genome. *Nucleic Acids Res.* **32,** D476–D481.

42. Eppig, J. T., Bult, C. J., Kadin, J. A., et al. (2005) The Mouse Genome Database (MGD): from genes to mice—a community resource for mouse biology. *Nucleic Acids Res.* **33,** D471–D475.

43. Bogue, M. (2003) Mouse Phenome Project: understanding human biology through mouse genetics and genomics. *J. Appl. Physiol.* **95,** 1335–1337.

44. Bogue, M. A. and Grubb, S. C. (2004) The Mouse Phenome Project. *Genetica* **122,** 71–74.

45. Schwartz, S., Kent, W. J., Smit, A., et al. (2003) Human-mouse alignments with BLASTZ. *Genome Res.* **13,** 103–107.

46. Brudno, M., Do, C. B., Cooper, G. M., et al. (2003) LAGAN and Multi-LAGAN: efficient tools for large-scale multiple alignment of genomic DNA. *Genome Res.* **13,** 721–731.

47. Brudno, M., Malde, S., Poliakov, A., et al. (2003) Glocal alignment: finding rearrangements during alignment. *Bioinformatics* **19(Suppl 1),** i54–i62.

48. Bray, N., Dubchak, I., and Pachter, L. (2003) AVID: a global alignment program. *Genome Res.* **13,** 97–102.

49. Blanchette, M., Kent, W. J., Riemer, C., et al. (2004) Aligning multiple genomic sequences with the threaded blockset aligner. *Genome Res.* **14,** 708–715.

50. Felsenstein, J. and Churchill, G. A. (1996) A Hidden Markov Model approach to variation among sites in rate of evolution. *Mol. Biol. Evol.* **13,** 93–104.

51. Siepel, A. and Haussler, D. (2004) Combining phylogenetic and hidden Markov models in biosequence analysis. *J. Comput. Biol.* **11,** 413–428.

52. Siepel, A. and Haussler, D. (2004) Phylogenetic estimation of context-dependent substitution rates by maximum likelihood. *Mol. Biol. Evol.* **21,** 468–488.

53. Schwartz, S., Zhang, Z., Frazer, K. A., et al. (2000) PipMaker—a web server for aligning two genomic DNA sequences. *Genome Res.* **10,** 577–586.

54. Elnitski, L., Riemer, C., Petrykowska, H., et al. (2002) PipTools: a computational toolkit to annotate and analyze pairwise comparisons of genomic sequences. *Genomics* **80,** 681–690.

55. Shah, N., Couronne, O., Pennacchio, L. A., et al. (2004) Phylo-VISTA: interactive visualization of multiple DNA sequence alignments. *Bioinformatics* **20,** 636–643.

56. Loots, G. G., Ovcharenko, I., Pachter, L., Dubchak, I., and Rubin, E. M. (2002) rVista for comparative sequence-based discovery of functional transcription factor binding sites. *Genome Res.* **12,** 832–839.

57. Loots, G. G. and Ovcharenko, I. (2004) rVISTA 2.0: evolutionary analysis of transcription factor binding sites. *Nucleic Acids Res.* **32,** W217–W221.

58. Boffelli, D., McAuliffe, J., Ovcharenko, D., et al. (2003) Phylogenetic shadowing of primate sequences to find functional regions of the human genome. *Science* **299,** 1391–1394.

59. Ovcharenko, I., Boffelli, D., and Loots, G. G. (2004) eShadow: a tool for comparing closely related sequences. *Genome Res.* **14,** 1191–1198.

60. Ovcharenko, I., Loots, G. G., Giardine, B. M., et al. (2005) Mulan: multiple-sequence local alignment and visualization for studying function and evolution. *Genome Res.* **15,** 184–194.

61. International HapMap Consortium. (2003) The International HapMap Project. *Nature* **426,** 789–796.

62. Giardine, B., Elnitski, L., Riemer, C., et al. (2003) GALA, a database for genomic sequence alignments and annotations. *Genome Res.* **13,** 732–741.

63. Elnitski, L., Giardine, B., Shah, P., et al. (2005) Improvements to GALA and dbERGE II: databases featuring genomic sequence alignment, annotation and experimental results. *Nucleic Acids Res.* **33,** D466–D470.

64. Camon, E., Barrell, D., Lee, V., Dimmer, E., and Apweiler, R. (2004) The Gene Ontology Annotation (GOA) Database—an integrated resource of GO annotations to the UniProt Knowledgebase. *In Silico. Biol.* **4,** 5–6.

65. Camon, E., Magrane, M., Barrell, D., et al. (2004) The Gene Ontology Annotation (GOA) Database: sharing knowledge in Uniprot with Gene Ontology. *Nucleic Acids Res.* **32,** D262–D266.

66. Harris, M. A., Clark, J., Ireland, A., et al. (2004) The Gene Ontology (GO) database and informatics resource. *Nucleic Acids Res.* **32,** D258–D261.

67. Cuff, J. A., Coates, G. M., Cutts, T. J., and Rae, M. (2004) The Ensembl computing architecture. *Genome Res.* **14,** 971–975.

68. Ashburner, M., Ball, C. A., Blake, J. A., et al. (2000) Gene ontology: tool for the unification of biology. The Gene Ontology Consortium. *Nat. Genet.* **25,** 25–29.

69. von Mering, C., Huynen, M., Jaeggi, D., Schmidt, S., Bork, P., and Snel, B. (2003) STRING: a database of predicted functional associations between proteins. *Nucleic Acids Res.* **31,** 258–261.

70. von Mering, C., Jensen, L. J., Snel, B., et al. (2005) STRING: known and predicted protein-protein associations, integrated and transferred across organisms. *Nucleic Acids Res.* **33,** D433–D437.

71. Brudno, M., Steinkamp, R., and Morgenstern, B. (2004) The CHAOS/DIALIGN WWW server for multiple alignment of genomic sequences. *Nucleic Acids Res.* **32,** W41–W44.

9

Positional Cloning

Single-Gene Cardiovascular Disorders

Duanxiang Li

Summary

Positional cloning is a comprehensive genetic strategy used to identify a disease-causing gene without any prior knowledge of the pathogenesis or protein defects involved in the disease process. The basic process involves collection of accurately diagnosed patients and their family members, genotyping DNAs with polymorphic DNA markers mapped to specific regions on chromosomes, genetic linkage analysis to determine markers that are in close proximity to the chromosome location of the disease gene and to define the critical region by haplotype analysis, identification and selection of candidate genes residing in the critical region, and, eventually, identification of the disease-causing DNA sequence variants by various methods. Many molecular techniques are utilized in positional cloning. Bioinformatics and computation analysis are significant and indispensable components of such a study, and are detailed elsewhere in this volume. This chapter presents a few basic laboratory protocols for conducting positional cloning: genomic DNA preparation, genotyping polymorphic markers, DNA sequencing, and related procedures that serve on fluorescent-labeled and capillary electrophoresis-based semi-automated genetic analysis systems.

Key Words: Positional cloning; cardiac disease; genotype; genetic marker; polymorphism; DNA sequence; mutation.

1. Introduction

It has been gradually but increasingly recognized by clinicians and patients alike that numerous cardiovascular diseases are inheritable. Many of them are monogenic disorders inherited in Mendelian fashion *(1,2)*. Examples of these diseases are familial hypercholesteromia, many forms of familial arrhythmia (Long Q-T syndrome, Brugada syndrome, familial atrial fibrillation, Wolf-Parkinson-White syndrome), various forms of familial cardiomyopathy

From: *Methods in Molecular Medicine, Vol. 128: Cardiovascular Disease; Methods and Protocols; Volume 1*
Edited by: Q. Wang © Humana Press Inc., Totowa, NJ

(hypertrophic, dilated, restrictive, and right ventricular cardiomyopathy), and some congenital heart defects. In just about 20 yr since the early discovery that mutations in the low-density lipoprotein receptor (LDLR) gene cause familial hypercholesteromia *(3)*, for instance, many genes have been successfully identified thanks largely to a widely used "positional cloning" strategy *(4–6)*. Consequently, our understanding, diagnosis, and management of these disorders have been greatly enhanced.

Positional cloning, or reverse genetics, as it was once referred to, is a comprehensive strategy used to identify a disease-causing gene without any prior knowledge of the pathogenesis or protein defects involved in the disease process *(7,8)*. The first and possibly most important step is to identify accurately diagnosed patients and their family members and to collect their blood or tissue samples for DNA extraction. The subjects' DNA samples are analyzed for polymorphic DNA markers at known chromosomal locations throughout the genome. These data are then used to determine which markers are inherited along with the disease trait in a given family. Markers that track through a family along with the disease trait are thought to be in close proximity (linked) to the disease gene. The critical region is defined as narrowly as possible by haplotype analysis. There may be dozens to hundreds of disease genes within the critical region, depending on its size and gene density. The next step is to evaluate these possible candidate genes based on what is known about their expression and function. Then, one must begin evaluating candidate genes for mutations in an effort to find the one that is disease-causing *(7)*. The strategy has been well established and greatly improved over the last decade by readily available, highly polymorphic markers; widely used PCR technology for both genotyping and DNA sequencing; semi-automated DNA analysis; and the much greater computing power that can be afforded to linkage analysis. However, a project aiming to identify a causal gene for cardiac diseases by positional cloning can still be very challenging. The challenges are due mostly to the complexity in defining a phenotype as well as the difficulty in selecting or finding the right candidate genes *(9,10)*.

Any segment of a DNA sequence can be used as a marker if it is polymorphic within the population and is informative for tracking down the genetic transmission. The most commonly used markers are thousands of simple sequence-length polymorphisms (SSLPs) or short tandem repeats (STRs), also known as microsatellites. They are DNA sequences with variable numbers of di-, tri-, or tetranucleotide repeats. The dinucleotide (CA) repeats are particularly abundant throughout the eukaryotic genome. These markers are highly informative, have been extensively characterized *(11)*, and can be readily genotyped by PCR *(12,13)*. Several detection methods, such as autoradiography, silver staining, and chemiluminescence, have been widely used to assess the PCR amplified products (alleles). For most of high-throughput applications, fluorescence-based genotyping has become standard technology *(14)*.

As the Human Genome Project is completed and most of genes are annotated, the number of genes that might be screened can be daunting even within a relatively small critical interval. A thoughtful selection on all candidate genes mapped in the region can greatly improve efficiency. Unfortunately, there is no definite rule one can apply to conducting such a selection, because there is a lack of knowledge of the biological or biochemical nature of numerous cardiovascular diseases, which is often the precise reason for pursuing the positional cloning strategy. Several guiding ideas, however, have proven quite helpful in selecting candidate genes for cardiovascular genetic diseases. Most of the genes identified so far as being responsible for adult cardiac diseases, for instance dilated and hypertrophic cardiomyopathy, are highly or preferentially expressed in hearts *(1,15)*; numerous genetically engineered animal models have provided important clues in finding human disease-causing genes with similar phenotypes *(16,17)*. Thus, gene expression profiles and the possible functions of a gene based on in vivo or in vitro experiments should be carefully considered in the context of potential or suspected pathogenesis of the diseases under investigation. Should a DNA variation be revealed by sequencing, a tentative disease-causing mutation can be distinguished from a benign polymorphism by its cosegaregation with the disease in the family; its absence in large number (minimum of 100) of unaffected and ethnically matched but unrelated individuals; change in a conserved amino acid within a conserved protein domain or region; and any functional consequence predicted or observed.

Many molecular techniques are being utilized in positional cloning. A comprehensive coverage of these topics is far beyond the scope of this chapter. It should be noted that bioinformatics and computation analysis are significant and indispensable components of such a study, and are discussed in detail elsewhere in this volume. This chapter focuses on the most frequently utilized and basic laboratory methods for conducting positional cloning: genomic DNA preparation, genotyping, DNA sequencing, and related methods (*see* **Note 1**). Among a wide range of methods with which genotyping and sequencing can be performed, from Southern blotting to manual polyacrylamide gel electrophoresis to microarray DNA chip technology, fluorescent-labeled and capillary electrophoresis-based semi-automated genetic analysis methods have become the mainstay in most research-oriented laboratories with moderate to high throughput *(14,18)*. These methods are described in detail here.

2. Materials

2.1. Genomic DNA Extraction From Whole Blood

1. Red cell lysis buffer: 0.32 M sucrose, 10 mM Tris-HCl, pH 7.5, 5 mM MgCl$_2$, 1% (v/v) Triton X-100.
2. Nuclear lysis buffer: 400 mM NaCl, 0.5% sodium dodecyl sulfate (SDS), 10 mM Tris-HCl, pH 8.0, 1 mM EDTA, pH 8.0.
3. Protenase K: dilute to 10 mg/mL in water. Aliquot and store at –20°C. It can be stored at 4°C for a few weeks.
4. Saturated NaCl: approx 6 M.

2.2. PCR and Genotyping

1. Subjects' DNA at a concentration of 10 ng/μL.
2. 4 dNTP mix, 2.5 mM.
3. 25 mM MgCl$_2$.
4. Fluorochrome-labeled forward primer for a DNA marker, 5 μM.
5. Reverse primer for a DNA marker, 5 μM.
6. AmpliTaq Gold DNA polymerase, 5 U/μL (Applied Biosystems).
7. 10X PCR Gold Buffer (Applied Biosystems).
8. Deionized formamide.
9. Fluorochrome-labeled DNA size Standard (ROX 500 or LIZ500 from Applied Biosystems, or others).
10. 96-well PCR plates (GeneMate).
11. Thermal adhesive sealing film for PCR (Fisher Scientific).
12. Multichannel pipettor, 8 or 12 channels of P10.
13. Thermal cyclers: the GeneAmp PCR System 9700 or any other systems.

2.3. DNA Sequencing

1. BigDye terminator (Applied Biosytems).
2. Sequencing buffer (Applied Biosytems).
3. PCR product presequencing kit (exonuclease I [*Exo*I] 10 U/μL and shrimp alkaline phosphatase 2 U/μL, product of USB).
4. MultiScreen Column Loader, 45 μL (Millipore).
5. Sephadex G-50 Superfine (Sigma or Amershan Pharmacia Biotech).
6. Multiscreen filter plate (Millipore).
7. ABI PRISM 3100 Genetic Analyzer (Applied Biosytems).

3. Methods

The fluorescent-based genotyping described in this section uses ABI 3100 Genetic Analyzer (Applied Biosystems), but it can be adapted to many other similar systems. For a whole genome scan, investigators normally opt to use a commercially available genetic mapping set. The set consists of well-optimized polymorphic DNA makers designed to cover the whole genome with specified density (from every 2.5–20 cM). To target a specific chromosome region, one can order fluorescent-labeled customer primers from any of the major oligonucleotide suppliers.

PCR is carried out to amplify the polymorphic markers with primers labeled with different fluorescent chemicals (FAM, HEX, TET, NED, and so on) and DNA from subjects. The fluorescent-labeled PCR products, excited by a laser when they pass through the capillary by electrophoresis, are detected by a sensor within the Genetic Analyzer. Because the Genetic Analyzer can differentiate the sizes and the color of each PCR product, DNA markers of different size (normally between 100 and 350 bp) labeled with three different colors (normally blue, green, and yellow) of the same subject's DNA are pooled for multiplex analysis. The data are collected automatically by computer and analyzed initially by Genescan (Applied Biosystems). The alleles are then called by the Genotyper program. When validated by experienced personnel, these allele data are ready for linkage calculation.

Once a critical chromosome region is defined by linkage and haplotype analysis, a list of positional candidate genes can be compiled and selected. Many mutation-screen and detection techniques can be used depending on the nature of the mutations. Disease-causing mutations (such as large insertions, deletions, inversions, and duplications) can grossly alter the gene structure. Cytogenetic study, Southern blot hybridization, restriction mapping, and pulsed-field gel electrophoresis have been successfully used to assess such gross changes.

The majority of the mutations, however, are caused by minimal changes in gene sequences such as missense mutations, small insertions, and small deletions, and a very different set of techniques are required to identify these mutations *(19)*. Most mutation screening methods are based on the following: mutated DNA fragments adopt different conformation; or heteroduplex formed between normal and mutant DNA molecules have different mobility or can be cleaved by specific chemicals or nucleases. The commonly used methods include single-strand conformational polymorphism (SSCP), chemical cleavage, denaturing gradient gel electrophoresis (DGGE), and denaturing high-performance liquid chromatography (dHPLC). Apart from being technically demanding, these methods do not offer the desired high sensitivity and specificity, as does positional cloning. Even if a mutation is detected, its nature cannot be revealed by these screening methods. Therefore, DNA sequencing is required in order to determine the exact nature of the mutation. An advantage for most of these screening methods is high efficiency. Hundreds or thousands of samples can be quickly screened in a matter of days after the optimal conditions are established.

Direct DNA sequence analysis has long been the gold standard for detecting point mutations, small insertions and deletions because of its high sensitivity and specificity. As the technology has been dramatically advanced, it is now possible to carry out a large number of DNA sequencing reactions with high efficiency and reasonable cost. Consequently, direct DNA sequencing is becoming the preferred method for mutation searches *(20)*. With this method, PCR-amplified patients' DNA fragments are directly sequenced and the precise nature of the mutation is revealed, provided the right candidate gene is under investigation.

3.1. Isolation of DNA From Whole Blood or Cultured Cells by Salting Out Method (21) (see Note 2)

Begin with whole blood anticoagulated with ACD or EDTA and a PBS-washed cell pellet.

1. Pour contents of one vacutainer (~10 mL) into a 50-mL conical tube. Add red cell lysis buffer to 50 mL. Mix by inversion and centrifuge at 1300g (2500 rpm on Sorvall RT-6000B with swinging bucket) for 15 min.
2. Pour off (or aspirate) about 42 mL supernatant. Resuspend pellet, pour into a 15-mL conical tube, fill tube with red cell lysis buffer, and recentrifuge as described previously.
3. Pour off supernatant, being careful not to disturb the pellet.
4. Resuspend cell pellet in 3 mL nuclear lysis buffer Add 75 µL protenase K (6 mL nuclear lysis buffer and 100 µL of protenase K is needed for >10^7 cells). Mix by inversion.
5. Incubated at 56°C for 1 h and 37°C for 6 h to overnight.
6. Add 1 mL of saturated NaCl for each 3 mL of nuclear lysis buffer used in **step 4**. Shake vigorously. Centrifuge at 1300g for 15 min to pellet protein and cell debris.
7. Remove supernatant to a new tube (15 or 50 mL, depending on the amount of supernatant). Add two volumes of room-temperature absolute ethanol. Mix by inversion. A cottony precipitate forms; this is nucleic acid.
8. Centrifuge the precipitate for 5 min at 1900g (3000 rpm on Sorvall RT-6000B with swinging bucket). Decant the supernatant.
9. Add 5 mL of 70% ethanol to wash the pellet, and centrifuge the precipitate for 5 min at 1900g. Decant the ethanol. Completely drain the tube and dry the pellet briefly.
10. Dissolve the DNA with 500 µL TE, pH 8.0 at 37°C for 2 h or longer. Now, the DNA is ready for quantification and usage (*see* **Note 3**).

3.2. PCR Amplification of DNA Markers From Subjects' Genomic DNA

1. For each PCR reaction of a total volume of 10 µL, the following reagents are needed (*see* **Note 4**):

H_2O	2.4 μL
PCR Gold buffer	1.0 μL
$MgCl_2$ (25 mM)	1.0 μL
dNTP mix	1.0 μL
Primer mix	0.5 μL
Amplitaq Gold	0.1 μL
DNA template	4.0 μL

2. Seal the tubes with caps or plates with appropriate sealing films. Briefly vortex and spin down the tubes or plates. Place the PCR reaction in a thermocycler and start the reaction with following cycling conditions on PE9700.

Initial activation:	94°C for 12 min
15 cycles:	94°C for 15 s
	55°C for 30 s
	72°C for 30 s
20 cycles:	90°C for 15 s
	55°C for 30 s
	72°C for 30 s
Final extension:	72°C for 15 min
Hold:	4°C

3.3. Pooling of Genotyping PCR Products Preparation of Genotyping Samples for Capillary Electrophoresis

1. Two important principles must be considered: first, only genotyping PCR products from the same DNA template can be pooled and to be differentiated by their distinguishable sizes and colors on the Genetic Analyzer; second, different ABI filter sets dictate the combination of the fluorochrome that can be used as listed next:

ABI 3100/DS-30/filter set D:	HEX/FAM/NED/ROX
ABI 3100/DS-31/filter set D:	VIC/FAM/NED/ROX
ABI 3100/DS-33/Filter set G5:	VIC/FAM/NED/LIZ

2. To make the size standard solution, add 1 μL of ROX (or others) to each 12 μL of deionized formide, mix well, and spin. Aliquot 12 μL of above size standard solution to each well of a 96-well plate.
3. Take 4 μL of genotyping products from the same DNA (normally PCR amplified with different markers of the same panel) into a pool (*see* **Note 5**); mix them well and spin.
4. Transfer 2 μL of the original or diluted pooled genotyping samples to each well that has been preloaded with a size standard:

   Panels with ≥10 markers, transfer the original pooled samples.
   Panels with 5–10 markers, transfer 1:1 diluted pooled samples.
   Panels with <5 markers, transfer 1:2 diluted pooled samples.

5. Denature the above samples at 94°C for 5 min; now, samples are ready to load onto the ABI 3100 for processing.

3.4. PCR Amplification of Candidate Gene From Patient's Genomic DNA

1. For a single reaction of 20 μL, add the following reagents per reaction:

dH$_2$O	9.9 μL
dNTP (2.5 mM)	1.0 μL
10X PCR Gold Buffer	2.0 μL
MgCl$_2$ (25 mM)	2.0 μL
AmpliTaq Gold (5 U/μL)	0.1 μL
Forward primer (5 μM)	0.5 μL
Reverse primer (5 μM)	0.5 μL
DNA (10 ng/μL)	4.0 μL

2. Seal the tubes with caps or plates with appropriate sealing films. Briefly vortex and spin down the tubes or plates. Place the PCR reaction in a thermocycler and start the reaction with following touch-down cycling conditions (*see* **Note 6**) on PE9700.

Initial activation:	94°C 12 min
10 cycles:	94°C for 15 s
	65°C for 30 s, decreasing by 1°C/cycle
	72°C for 45 s
30 cycles:	90°C for 15 s
	55°C for 30 s
	72°C for 45 s
Final extension:	72°C for 5 min
Hold:	4°C forever

3.5. Purification of PCR Products With ExoI-SAP Enzymatic Method (see Note 7)

1. Dilute *Exo*I and shrimp alkaline phosphatase (SAP) with 1X the same PCR buffer/ MgCl$_2$ used for PCR (1 μL of each enzymes to 2 μL of 1X PCR buffer with MgCl$_2$).
2. Set up the reaction as following:

PCR product	5 μL
ExoI/SAP (diluted)	2 μL

3. Perform the reaction on thermocycler: 37°C for 40 min followed by 80°C for 15 min. Take 3.0 μL of the products to run sequencing reactions.

3.6. Performing Cycling Sequencing Reactions With BigDye Terminator Reaction

1. For a single reaction of 20 μL, add the following reagents per reaction (*see* **Note 8**):

dH$_2$O	12.0 μL
5X buffer	2.0 μL
BigDye terminators	2.0 μL
Primer (5 m*M*, forward OR reverse)	1.0 μL
PCR product (10–30 ng, purified)	3.0 μL

Mix well and spin down briefly.

2. Cycling sequencing using PCR Products on thermocyclers:

30 cycles:	96°C for 10 s
	50°C for 5 s
	60°C for 120 s
Hold:	4°C

3.7. Clean Up the Sequencing Extension Products Using MultiScreen 96-Well Filtration Plates for Electrophoresis (see Note 9)

1. Load dry Sephadex G-50 (Sigma) Superfine onto a 45-mL, 96-well multiscreen loader and remove the excessive resin from the top of the column using a Plexiglas plate.
2. Move the Sephadex into a new Multiscreen Clear (column) plate by fitting in and inverting the plates.
3. Hydrate the Sephadex by adding 300 mL of Milli-Q water to each well and incubate at room temperature for 3 h.
4. Centrifuge at 1200*g* for 3 min (2400 rpm on Sorvall tabletop centrifuge) with any regular plate as liquid collector.
5. Replace the bottom plate with a clean 96-well plate for ABI 3100.
6. Transfer 20 mL of labeled sequencing reaction products to center of each well.
7. Centrifuge at 1200*g* for 5 min.
8. Dry the product with speed vacuum AND then reconstitute them with 10 mL of H$_2$O.
9. Denature at 90°C for 2 min and cool them with ice water immediately, then dry the plate and load it onto ABI 3100 sample tray. Samples are ready for electrophoresis and analysis on the Genetic Analyzer.

4. Notes

1. The protocols for PCR and sequencing reactions presented here are based on a single reaction. The user can easily scale up the number of reactions to run. To make a master mixture for a plate of 96 reactions, a factor of 100 works well.
2. The salting out protocol is cost-effective and simple way to extract high quality DNA from larger volume (10 mL or more) of whole blood. The yield is 10–20 μg DNA from 1 mL of whole blood. The DNA can be used for almost all molecular biology applications. There are numerous other methods, including commercial kits and DNA extraction machines. Investigators can choose suitable methods for their experimental purposes.

3. For short-term storage or diluted working solution, DNA can be placed at 4°C. For long-term storage, DNA can be stored at –20°C or –80°C if it is to be used for PCR amplification. The same principle can apply to oligonucleotides used for primers.

4. PCR is a versatile and powerful in vitro DNA cloning method. Because of its high sensitivity to contamination, every care must exercised not to introduce any DNA other than those templates intended for the reaction. Practical rules include: perform PCR in a separate bench area with dedicated pipetors; always wear gloves; change the tips whenever it is necessary; always include a negative control; and if available, run a positive control, because this might help in troubleshooting. The condition listed in this protocol shall serve as a start-up protocol. It can be modified in many ways, mostly depending on the target DNA sequence, primers, Taq polymerase to be used, and thermal cyclers. For the thermal cyclers without a hot-top, a few drops of mineral oil should be added on the top of PCR reaction to prevent evaporation.

5. The relative intensity of dye labels varies, and their use depends on the mode of the filter to be used. FAM has relative high intensity, whereas TET has quite a low intensity. The yield of the PCR reaction can be quite variable. The optimal relative intensity for ABI Genetic Analyzer is in the range of 200 to 2000. Too low an intensity may lose alleles; too high an intensity, particularly those >4000, can result in serious bleed through into other spectral channels, thus introducing errant alleles. Thus, the appropriate ration for pooling the genotyping products deserve careful consideration. Many investigators check the genotyping products on agarose gels and adjust the amount to be pooled according to the yield. We normally accomplish this calibration through careful PCR condition tests so that different markers produce a roughly equal amount of products. Equal pooling methods have worked well in the author's laboratory.

6. Effective use of hot-start and touchdown PCR has nearly eliminated the need to optimize PCR conditions, and, thus, proven to be cost-effective.

7. PCR products must be verified by visualizing on an agarose gel. PCR products can be purified by many different procedures. The PCR extraction kit (from Qiagen or other manufacturers) and gel extraction are two widely used methods. Use of the enzymatic methods (the *Exo*I to remove residual single-stranded primers and shrimp alkaline phosphatase to remove the remaining dNTPs from PCR mixture) has proven to be simple and effective. It is the preferred method in our laboratory.

8. The manufacturer's sequencing protocol works fine, but is very costly and time consuming. We did a series of tests and made some significant modifications. Described here is a somewhat modified and very robust protocol for sequencing PCR products.

9. Precipitation methods employing ethanol to remove unincorporated dye terminator are more likely to be incomplete and, thus, obscure the beginning of the sequence. Many spin columns or filtration kits are commercially available. The protocol described here is reliable and cost-effective for performing for large

numbers of sequences. The hydrated multiscreen filtration plates can be stored in a refrigerator if they are sealed in a plastic bag with a water-saturated paper towel within in order to keep them moist.

References

1. Wang, Q., Chen, Q., and Towbin, J. A. (1998) Genetics, molecular mechanisms and management of long QT syndrome. *Ann. Med.* **30**, 58–65.
2. Brugada, R., Brugada, J., and Roberts, R. (1999) Genetics of cardiovascular disease with emphasis on atrial fibrillation. *J. Interv. Card. Electrophysiol.* **3**, 7–13.
3. Lehrman, M. A., Goldstein, J. L., Brown, M. S., Russell, D. W., and Schneider, W. J. (1985) Internalization-defective LDL receptors produced by genes with nonsense and frameshift mutations that truncate the cytoplasmic domain. *Cell* **41**, 735–743.
4. Roberts, R. (2000) A perspective: the new millennium dawns on a new paradigm for cardiology —molecular genetics. *J. Am. Coll. Cardiol.* **36**, 661–667.
5. Semsarian, C. and Seidman, C. (2001) Molecular medicine in the 21st century. *Internal Medicine Journal* **31**, 53–59.
6. Burkett, E. L. and Hershberger, R. E. (2005) Clinical and genetic issues in familial dilated cardiomyopathy. *J. Am. Coll. Cardiol.* **45**, 969–981.
7. Roberts, R. (1992) *Molecular Basis of Cardiology,* Blackwell Scientific Hamden, CT, pp.15–112.
8. Schofield, P. R. (2001) Genetics, an alternative way to discover, characterize and understand ion channels. *Clin. Exp. Pharmacol. Physiol.* **28**, 84–88.
9. Morita, H., Seidman, J., and Seidman, C. (2005) Genetic causes of human heart failure. *J. Clin. Invest.* **115**, 518–526.
10. Lusis, A.J. (2003) Genetic factors in cardiovascular disease. 10 questions. *Trends Cardiovasc. Med.* **13**, 09–316.
11. Kong, A., Gudbjartsson, D. F., Sainz, J., et al. (2002) A high-resolution recombination map of the human genome. *Nat. Genet.* **31**, 241–247.
12. Weber, J. L. and May, P. E. (1989) Abundant class of human DNA polymorphisms which can be typed using the polymerase chain reaction. *Am. J. Hum. Genet.* **44**, 388–396.
13. Litt, M. and Luty, J.A. (1989) A hypervariable microsatellite revealed by in vitro amplification of a dinucleotide repeat within the cardiac muscle actin gene. *Am. J. Hum. Genet.* **44**, 397–401.
14. Ziegle, J. S., Su, Y., Corcoran, K. P., et al. (1992) Application of automated DNA sizing technology for genotyping microsatellite loci. *Genomics* **14**, 1026–1031.
15. Li, D., Czernuszewicz, G., Gonzalez, O., et al. (2001) Dilated cardiomyopathy caused by a novel mutation in cardiac troponin T gene. *Circulation* **104**, 2188–2193.
16. Li, D., Tapscoft, T., Gonzalez, O., et al. (1999) Desmin mutation responsible for idiopathic dilated cardiomyopathy. *Circulation* **100**, 461–464.
17. McKoy, G., Protonotarios, N., Crosby, A., et al. (2000) Identification of a deletion in plakoglobin in arrhythmogenic right ventricular cardiomyopathy with palmoplantar keratoderma and woolly hair (Naxos disease). *Lancet* **355**, 2119–2124.

18. Graham, C. A. and Hill, A. J. (2001) Fluorescent sequencing for heterozygote mutation detection. *Methods Mol. Biol.* **167,** 193–213.
19. Mashal, R. D. and Sklar, J. (1996) Practical methods of mutation detection. *Curr. Opin. Genet. Dev.* **6,** 275–280.
20. Taylor, C. F. and Taylor, G. R. (2004) Current and emerging techniques for diagnostic mutation detection: an overview of methods for mutation detection. *Methods Mol. Med.* **92,** 9–44.
21. Miller, S. A., Dykes, D. D., and Polesky, H. F. (1988) A simple salting out procedure for extracting DNA from human nucleated cells. *Nucleic Acids Res.* **16,** 1215.

10

Positional Cloning

Complex Cardiovascular Traits

Jeffery Gulcher and Kari Stefansson

Summary

Cardiovascular traits represent the quintessential complex trait derived from the confluence of numerous genetic and environmental risk factors. Therefore, positional cloning of cardiovascular genes contributing to the common forms of cardiovascular disease is much more challenging than the mapping and isolation of genes contributing to rare Mendelian phenocopies of cardiovascular disease. Success requires careful and systematic phenotyping, large numbers of families that contain multiple patients, and high-quality genotyping covering for both genome scan and the follow-up case–control association study testing the genes and LD blocks within the linkage peaks.

Key Words: Linkage; genotyping; microsatellites; single-nucleotide polymorphisms; SNPs; positional cloning.

1. Introduction

Positional cloning through linkage analysis is a genetic mapping approach that relies on families, each with more than one individual with a particular disease phenotype. Markers covering the entire genome are used to genotype patients and unaffected family members, and the method looks for segments of the genome in patients that are identical-by-descent (shared) in excess of what is expected by chance or that cosegregate with the disease. Although the candidate gene approach is valuable, linkage analysis has several advantages that complement it:

1. It is hypothesis-independent and allows for the possibility of finding something unanticipated—this is a particularly important advantage in a disease as compli-

From: *Methods in Molecular Medicine, Vol. 128: Cardiovascular Disease; Methods and Protocols; Volume 1*
Edited by: Q. Wang © Humana Press Inc., Totowa, NJ

cated and multifactorial as myocardial infarction (MI).

2. It is a cost-effective method for scanning the entire genome because it requires a smaller number of markers and much less dramatic correction of the *p* value than would be required for a whole-genome association scan.

3. It provides a way to scan the entire genome and prioritize the regions that contain disease genes with strongest effect—linkage cannot detect genes with minimal or modest effect on the disease—therefore, significant linkage peaks, if present, may map genes that have a more substantial effect on disease risk.

4. Including multiple patients related to common ancestors in each family may represent a way to link together patients who are more likely to share the same biological and genetic basis for their disease.

Several linkage scans have been reported for cardiovascular and related diseases. The phenotypes used in the patients including in the linkage scan are cardiovascular events (MI or stroke), procedural correction of significant atherosclerosis (peripheral arterial occlusive disease), arterial thickness (such as carotid intimal-medial thickness [IMT]), and risk factors for cardiovascular disease such as type 1 and type 2 diabetes, hypertension, hypercholesterolemia, obesity, and smoking history. The following describes the linkage approach that we have practiced in Iceland to map and isolate genes for cardiovascular disease including *FLAP*, *PDE4D*, and *EP3* *(1–4)*.

2. Materials

2.1. Phenotyping

The materials for clinical phenotyping are specific to the cardiovascular parameters selected for the genetics study.

2.2. Ascertainment of Families

1. Pedigree drawing and management software such as Progeny 5 (Progeny Software, LLC, South Bend, IN) (www.progeny2000.com).

2. A software package that uses genotypes to check relationships between pairs of individuals in the same pedigree such as Relatedness 5.0 (http://www.gsoftnet.us/GSoft.html) or Broman and Weber's modification of Relcheck (http://www.biostat.jhsph.edu/~kbroman/software/).

2.3. Collection and Storage of Blood

Plastic 10-mL vacutainers with EDTA (BD plastic vacutainer blood tubes with EDTA; Becton Dickinson, Co, Franklin Lakes, NJ; cat. no. 366643).

2.4. Isolation of DNA From Blood

Flexigene DNA isolation kit (Qiagen, Valencia, CA; cat. no. 51204).

2.5. Genome-Wide Microsatellite Genotyping

1. Liquid handling by high-speed low-volume robotics such as Sciclone ALH 3000 Workstation (Caliper, Hopkinton, MA).
2. ABI 3730 Capillary DNA Analyzer (Applied Biosystems, Foster City, CA).
3. Allele calling by GeneMapper 4.0 (Applied Biosystems).
4. PCR reagents such as Amplitaq Gold (Applied Biosystems).
5. Fluorescent labeled PCR primers (Applied Biosystems).
6. Thermal cyclers such as DNA Engines from MJ Research, Waltham, MA.

2.6. Linkage Analysis

Linkage analysis software such as Allegro, Decode Genetics, Reykjavik, Iceland (www.decode.com) or SOLAR (*see* Chapter 7), SimWalk, GENEHUNTER or SAGE (*see* Chapter 6).

2.7. Follow-Up Intermediate Fine-Mapping to Support Linkage Signal

See **Subheadings 2.5.** and **2.6.**

2.8. Hypothesis-Independent Ultrafine Mapping of Linkage Peaks and Case–Control Association

1. Case–control haplotype association software such as NEMO (www.decode.com) or MENDEL 5 (http://www.genetics.ucla.edu/software/mendel5) or PHASE (http://www.stat.washington.edu/stephens/).
2. High-throughput single-nucleotide polymorphism (SNP) methods such as Taqman (Applied Biosystems) or pyrosequencing or mass spectroscopy.

3. Methods

3.1. Phenotyping

High-quality phenotyping is essential in any genetic study. In cardiovascular disease, the three major categories for phenotyping are cardiovascular events, measurements of atherosclerosis, and risk factors. The most commonly ascertained cardiovascular events are MI or acute coronary syndrome event, stroke, revascularization procedure for coronary artery disease (CAD), carotid endarterectomy, revascularization procedure for symptomatic peripheral artery disease (PAD), measurements of atherosclerosis, and determination of risk factors. Note that events such as stroke have a long list of subtypes that are useful to obtain in greater detail. Measures of atherosclerosis include percentage stenosis by atherosclerosis plaques and the number of coronary blood vessels significantly involved in the coronary vasculature as assessed by coronary angiography. Newer methods such as intravascular ultrasound (IVUS) may directly measure thickness of coronary atherosclerosis plaques. The luminal dimension (degree of stenosis) of the common and internal carotids are usually assessed by ultrasound, magnetic resonance angiography (MRA), or carotid angiography. Carotid IMT measurements may also be made with the noninvasive methods of ultrasound and MRA. Carotid wall thickness, if measured accurately, appears to correlate with future cardiovascular events in some studies *(5,6)* and so is used by some in younger individuals as a surrogate for future significant atherosclerotic lesions and events. The advantage is that a larger number of people can be more conveniently included in the study, and the downside is that it represents an imperfect surrogate of the cardiovascular events that one is trying to study. Finally, there are a large number of medical and environmental risk factors for cardiovascular disease such as hypertension, hypercholesterolemia, diabetes, smoking, and obesity. Demographic data such as sex and age-of-onset of the events or measurements is also important to catalog in order to allow for genetic analysis of subphenotypes, such as early-onset MI and stroke in females.

3.2. Ascertainment of Families

A large number of families that have at least two affected relatives is necessary for a linkage study of any complex trait. It is important to have accurate information on relationships of the affected individuals within family. In affected-only nonparametric analysis, the most common approach used in linkage studies for common diseases, it is not necessary to have information on the relatives who are not going to be designated as affecteds; even if normal, they may later develop a cardiovascular event. Their phenotypes will be designated as "unknown" and will not be used. Instead, their genotypes will be used only to help derive the allelic sharing statistic between affecteds within the family. Therefore, collection of additional "unaffected" relatives who are closely related (first- or second-degree relatives) to the affecteds in the family can provide useful information if genotyped.

It is also important to prove the accuracy of the family structure. For example, it is not uncommon to find that a pair of siblings are actually half-siblings. Inaccuracies in the relationships can be flagged by applying relationship and inheritance checks on the genotype data from each family. A relationship check compares the number of alleles over several markers shared between the two individuals tested. For example, it is expected that full siblings will share 50% of their alleles, whereas a half-sibling pair will share 25%. Carrying out these checks with a panel of 10–20 microsatellites at the beginning of the study is useful to detect laboratory errors before creating the final DNA plates for the genome-wide genotyping.

3.3. Collection and Storage of Blood

Most methods for DNA isolation work best with blood samples that have been collected in EDTA-containing vacutainers that prevent blood coagulation. The standard size of vacutainers used in adult medicine can contain 8–10 mL of whole blood. It is prudent to collect the blood in plastic vacutainers rather than glass to decrease the chance of tube cracking on expansion of the blood in the freezer. It is important to store the blood frozen in such a way to prevent multiple freeze–thaw cycles. A well insulated freezer at –20°C or lower and that is not frost-free is most cost-effective. Such freezers can be obtained from most commodity freezer vendors in the United States. Many freezers available outside the United States are not well insulated and have difficulty maintaining or even achieving the necessary temperature. It is important to keep sample tubes within cardboard or plastic boxes to decrease impact of opening and closing the freezer door. A –80°C freezer is not necessary for sample storage and is much more expensive. However, its major benefit is that there should not be much of a risk for freeze–thaw unless the freezer itself fails. A sample tracking and laboratory information management system (LIMS) is important for any medium- or high-throughput lab (*see* **Note 1**).

3.4. Isolation of DNA From Blood

There are many suitable methods for isolation of DNA from whole blood. However, it should be emphasized that most (if not all) of the robotic methods currently available for DNA isolation from freshly collected blood do not work well for samples that are thawed from frozen blood. One reliable method for isolation of large quantities of high-quality DNA from a large volume of frozen blood (4–12 mL) is Qiagen's Flexigene kit (described as follows) for 10 mL of blood (adjust for actual volume), which routinely yields at least 250–350 µg of DNA from a frozen tube of blood:

1. Quick-thaw a frozen whole blood vacutainer tube in a gently shaking water bath of 37°C and store on ice until **step 2**.
2. Place 25 mL Buffer FG1 into a 50-mL centrifuge tube and add 10 mL of whole blood. Mix by inverting tube five times.
3. Centrifuge 5 min at 2000*g* in a swing-out rotor.
4. Discard supernatant and carefully drain inverted tube on clean paper towel for 2 min.
5. Add 5 mL Buffer FG2 with 50 µL of protease stock and vortex immediately until the pellet is completely lysed (very important).
6. Invert tube three times and incubate in water bath at 65°C for 10 min.

7. Add 5 mL of 100% isopropanol and mix by inversion until DNA precipitate becomes visible as threats or a clump.
8. Centrifuge for 3 min at 2000*g*.
9. Discard the supernatant and briefly invert tube onto clean paper towel making sure the pellet remains intact.
10. Add mL of 70% ethanol and vortex for 5 s.
11. Centrifuge for 3 min at 2000*g*.
12. Discard the supernatant and leave tube inverted on paper towel for at least 5 min and air-dry the DNA pellet until liquid drops have evaporated (at least 5 min). Do not overdry the pellet, or it may be difficult to resuspend.
13. Add 1 mL Buffer FG3, vortex for 5 s, and dissolve the DNA by incubating for 1 h at 65°C in a water bath.
14. Quantitate these concentrated DNA stocks using an ultraviolet spectrophotometer. If good quality by high A260 to A280 ratio and if it passes tests for PCR (we use a standard multiplex panel of 14 microsatellite markers, which represents a much more stringent quality test than nonpolymorphic DNA or SNPs), aliquot and store at –20°C. Keep a working stock at 4°C to prevent freeze–thaw breakdown of DNA.

3.5. Genome-Wide Microsatellite Genotyping

1. Design a 96-well DNA plate from a list of patients and relatives. Keeping most relatives together on a plate facilitates plate-by-plate inheritance checking for quality control. Place the DNA from a standard individual (such as the widely used CEPH individual 1347-02) into at least two of the wells to provide an internal plate check and to facilitate calibration across runs within the same laboratory and across laboratories.
2. Dilute the DNA into 750 µL of water or in 10 m*M* Tris, pH 7.5 to10 ng/µL. Place dilutions within deep-well 96-well plates.
3. As mentioned under **Subheading 3.4.**, the DNA is tested for quality and inheritance compatibility to relatives using a panel of 14 standard microsatellite markers before the samples proceed to additional SNP or microsatellite genotyping.
4. Quality control of the marker assays used in genetics projects is important. All subjects who are recruited for our genetics studies are genotyped either with Decode's 1200 microsatellite marker linkage set with fluorescently labeled primer sets or a 2000 microsatellite marker set, and so we have been able to develop a marker set with over 99.8% accuracy (based on inheritance checks covering more than 50 million genotypes). This microsatellite screening set is based in part on markers from the ABI Linkage Marker (v2) screening set and the ABI Linkage Marker (v2) intercalating set in combination with 800–1600 of our own custom-made markers and is widely available to any academic or commercial groups through Decode's Genotyping Service. All of these markers have been extensively tested for robustness, ease of scoring, and efficiency in 4X multiplex PCR reactions in the Icelandic and other populations, which is important for any genome-wide genotyping set. The location and genetic distances between

those 1200 markers have been accurately determined as a part of the Decode High Resolution Genetic Map. We constructed and made publicly available this genetic map by genotyping 869 volunteers, consisting of parents and offspring from 146 Icelandic families. This genetic map provides the relative order and location of 5136 microsatellite markers distributed across the whole genome and is considered by most to be the standard genetic map of the human genome (*see* National Center for Biotechnology Information [NCBI] and the University of California at Santa Cruz [UCSC] genome websites and Kong et al., 2000 *[7]*).

5. Set up the PCR reactions using DNA from the deep-well patient plates and plating by quadruplicate into 384-well plates using liquid-handling robots (we use Caliper robots). The reaction volume used is 5 µL, and for each multiplex PCR reaction of four markers, 20 ng of genomic DNA is amplified in the presence of 2 pmol of each primer, 0.25 U AmpliTaq Gold, 0.2 m*M* dNTPs and 2.5 m*M* MgCl$_2$ (buffer supplied by manufacturer, ABI). The PCR conditions used are 95°C for 10 min, then 37 cycles of 15 s at 94°C, 30 s at 55°C, and 1 min at 72°C in a thermocycler (we use MJR Thermocyclers). PCR products of 10–16 different markers from the same patient are pooled using liquid handling robots (we use Hydra robotics), supplemented with an internal size standard, and resolved on Applied Biosystems model 3700 or 3730 Capillary Sequencers using Genescan v3.0 peak calling software.

6. Call the genotypes using allele-calling software to determine the genotype at each marker for each patient such as the ABI Genotyper software along with follow-up manual editing to improve accuracy and salvage difficult genotypes (we use the Decode Allele Caller software).

7. All genotypes should be quality controlled at several levels. Immediately after the automatic allele calls, potential technical problems should be flagged, such as PCR product sizes outside the expected marker windows, incorrect genotypes for the standard, and genotype mismatches between the standard individual placed at least twice on each plate. These should provide immediate alerts to the genotyping facility for correction and rerunning of the patient plate. Raw and curated genotypes are stored in a genotype database that automatically applies quality control measures including inheritance checks, histogram checks, Hardy-Weinberg deviation, relationship checks, plate-to-plate variation, and linkage disequilibrium (LD) checks of closely spaced markers (*see* **Note 2** for greater detail).

3.6. Linkage Analysis

1. Determine the affection status of all individuals in the families that have been genotyped. An affecteds-only strategy requires a setting of either "affected" or "unknown" for the rest.

2. Include only families that contain two or more affected individuals who share common ancestors. Exclude all other families. Create pedigree files, which gives the real or virtual parents for each individual in the family.

3. Create a genotype file for each individual that gives the genotype for each marker successfully genotyped.

4. Run linkage using a multipoint linkage program such as Allegro *(8)*. Allegro calculates nonparametric logarithm of the odds (lod) scores based on multipoint calculations. It calculates the statistical significance of excess sharing among related patients by applying nonparametric affected-only allele sharing methods, independent of any particular inheritance model *(8–10)*. The baseline linkage analysis uses the S_{pairs} scoring function, the exponential allele-sharing model, and a family-weighting scheme halfway on a log scale between weighting each affected pair equally and weighting each family equally. For a single genome-wide scan, a lod score of 3.7 or a single-test p value of 2×10^{-5} is the threshold for statistical significance: A lod score in excess of 2.3 or a single-test p value of 5×10^{-4} is considered suggestive for linkage. In both cases, we would expect information content in excess of 90% before drawing conclusions *(11)* (*see* **Subheading 3.8.**).

5. Allegro computes p values two different ways and it is customary to report the larger (less significant) one to be on the conservative side. The first p value is computed based on large sample theory; $Zlr = \sqrt{(2 \log_e (10) \text{ lod})}$ is approximately distributed as a standard normal distribution under the null hypothesis of no linkage *(9)*. Allegro computes a second p value by comparing the observed lod score with its complete data sampling distribution under the null hypothesis as previously described *(8)*. When a data set consists of more than a handful of families, these two p values tend to be very similar.

3.7. Follow-Up Intermediate Fine Mapping to Support Linkage Signal

1. Add extra microsatellite markers over the linkage peaks that are suggestive or significant in the initial linkage scan to increase the information content to maximize use of the families in the study. The information measure we use and is part of the Allegro program output was defined by Nicolae *(11)* and is closely related to a classical measure of information as previously described by Dempster and colleagues *(12)*. Information equals zero if the marker genotypes are completely uninformative and equals one if the genotypes determine the exact amount of allele sharing by descent among the affected individuals. For a study with only 50% information content (which is the typical for affected sibling pair study with only 350 microsatellite markers if parents are not genotyped), only half of the families would be contributing to the study. Therefore, much more information can be extracted and the large investment already made in the collection and phenotyping of patients would be more fully leveraged if extra markers are added to the linkage peaks to boost the information content to 90% or greater.

2. Select microsatellite markers that cover the linkage peaks to a density of 0.5–1.5 cM spacing. There are plenty of already validated microsatellite markers to achieve this density in almost all locations of the genome available from the set of 5145 markers used to create the Decode high-resolution genetic map, which

has an average density of 0.6 cM (*see* NCBI and UCSC genome websites). Marker orders and intermarker sex-averaged distances in the peak region are available from this map. Correct marker order is essential for multipoint linkage analysis, and lod scores are affected by the estimates of the intermarker genetic distances. By selecting markers from the Decode high resolution genetic map (*7*), the marker order and sex-averaged (and sex specific) intermarker genetic distances are already known and do not need to be interpolated.

3. Use these markers to genotype within entire width of suggestive and significant linkage peaks according to the methods under **Subheading 3.5.**
4. Repeat linkage analysis of the chromosomes with added markers together with the framework markers.

3.8. Hypothesis-Independent Ultrafine Mapping of Linkage Peaks and Case–Control Association

1. Select a locus to follow-up to isolate the disease-associated gene responsible for the linkage signal. Select either (1) a linkage peak that meets criteria for significant genome-wide linkage or (2) a suggestive linkage peak that has support with a significant or suggestive linkage peak from an independent set of families. The commonly used criteria for genome-wide significant to a level of only p value less than 0.05 is the Lander-Kruglyak criteria (*13*) which, based on simulations, has set a threshold of a single-test p value of less than 2×10^{-5}; this corresponds to a lod of about 3.7 but depends on the family structure. Formally, an even more stringent p value is required if multiple genetic inheritance models are used in a parametric modeling in the linkage analysis. A typical parametric linkage study can look at more than 100 models and therefore can lead to high rate of false-positive linkage. To avoid such a dramatic correction of the p value, it is perhaps more prudent to use a single nonparametric model. We use a single sharing method that does assume a particular inheritance model. Additional formal correction of the p value comes from adjusting for the number of phenotype models used in the linkage study, although many of the phenotypes used in a single study correlate with each other and many of the patients and families will overlap among the runs; therefore, the appropriate correction factor may not be as great. It is always best to define a limited number of phenotypes to apply to a particular cohort to limit this correction factor.
2. Select the method of follow-up: either (1) a candidate gene case–control association study or (2) a hypothesis-independent locus-wide case–control association study. The former has the advantage that it is much faster and cheaper. However, the danger of hypothesis testing in human genetics is that one may find subtle association to one of the candidate genes and may miss the strongest association signal under the linkage peak, which might reveal a more important pathway. Modern human genetics allows for more complete assessment in a genome-wide and locus-wide manner, allowing researchers to find some surprises. For example, no one had previously hypothesized and tested neuregulin 1 in the context of

schizophrenia or any other psychiatric conditions until Decode found linkage to chromosome 8p and tested all LD blocks under the linkage peak for association *(14)*. In fact, four other groups had already reported linkage to 8p and had tested numerous candidate genes but ignored neuregulin 1. Therefore, locus-wide association studies allow the researcher to keep an open mind and to have greater confidence that the association found is the strongest in the locus.

3. Determine the entire risk interval of the linkage peak that is to be assessed by extra markers. If the peak is significant and comes out of a linkage cohort with at least 400 patients within extended families we focus extra markers on the one-lod drop interval; that is, the segment defined by the a drop of one lod from the peak lod. However, for significant peaks from smaller studies or from suggestive peaks, it may be best to cover the two-lod drop interval.

4. Select the type and number of markers to be used in the association study. Some prefer to use only SNPs given their stability over generations, ease of genotyping, and the wealth of linkage-disequilibrium data, already available from the HapMap, on almost 300 people from diverse ethnic backgrounds (www.hapmap.org). The current average density of SNP coverage from HapMap is about 5 kb and will increase by the end of 2005. These data provide a measure of LD structure within any linkage peak and the selection of less redundant SNPs to cover each LD block. That is, if the average LD block in Caucasians is about 60 kb, then there are an average of 12 SNPs available from HapMap per LD block. Many SNPs will be in very tight LD with correlation with other SNPs in the block as assessed by r^2 greater than 0.95, and therefore are likely to be redundant in terms of information provided. Selection of 5 SNPx or more may capture the same amount of information as 12 SNPs—therefore, assessment of each LD block under the linkage peak may be faster and cheaper using TagSNPs. More cost-effective custom genotyping platforms are available now to facilitate genotyping the large number of markers and patients needed for such a study. The one-lod drop interval is generally smaller if extended families are used and the one-lod drop may average 4–7 cM (or approx 4–7 million bases for average region but depends on the local meiotic recombination rate). For studies with mainly affected sibling pairs, the intervals will be even larger. For an interval of 5 million bases, there are from 50 to 150 LD blocks and if five Tag-SNPs are used for each, then 250–750 SNP markers may be needed to cover the LD structure.

5. Select patient and control cohorts for case–control association. For common diseases, it is important to have a powered case–control study. For a locus-wide association study using almost 1000 markers, the *p* value of significant association when accounting for multiple marker testing will need to be smaller than 0.01 by a factor of 1000, perhaps more if haplotype association is tried. Therefore, the cohorts used for association should be at least 500 to 1000 individuals within each cohort, although a smaller number might be useful to find very common variants. For association studies that test the entire linkage peaks, sample sizes of 575 patients and 575 controls are needed to have 90% power to detect a variant of population allelic frequency 10% with a RR of 2.0 and nominal *p* value

of 10^{-5} (which may be necessary to account for multiple markers tested) (*see* **Note 3** for a table of power calculations for haplotype association).

6. Genotype the SNP markers in the selected cohorts using one of many available SNP platforms. For a genotyping 1000 or more SNPs per patient, it may be more cost-effective to use a custom-made bead or chip array platform. As discussed under **Subheading 3.5.**, quality control of genotyping is essential.

7. Assess and increase diversity of haplotypes. Using enough markers to define the LD structure of the candidate gene or linkage peak region is only part of the challenge. The other equally important factor in powering an association study is to define enough of the haplotype space within each LD block. Failure to have enough haplotype diversity in an LD block may lead to the situation in which the disease-associated functional variant is on the background of a very common ancestral haplotype. If the variant is only on a portion of the common haplotype then that haplotype may not show tight enough correlation to the disease and the gene association will be missed. That is, the haplotype was a poor surrogate for the underlying functional variant. To decrease that chance, it is best to assess haplotype diversity among all LD blocks and to attempt to further break up common haplotypes of frequency greater than 10–20% by added more SNP markers if available and not redundant with the previously used SNPs or adding microsatellite markers. We find that a combination of TagSNPs and the more much more informative microsatellite markers increases the haplotype diversity within most LD blocks beyond what can be achieved even if genotyping all available HapMap SNPs. There are plenty of polymorphic microsatellites to be able to be genotype at least one per LD block. The mutation rate of microsatellites (which averages 5×10^{-4} per generation) is high enough to split up ancestral SNP haplotypes and low enough to represent stable surrogates for underlying functional variants (*see* **Note 4** for selection of new microsatellite markers). The density we aim for is to have on average one marker every 12 kb requiring about 400 SNP and microsatellite markers (we usually use about 250 TagSNPs from the HapMap dataset and 150 microsatellite markers per linkage peak). It is straightforward to integrate microsatellite markers into the LD patterns. In this analysis, the standard definitions of D' and R^2 are extended to include microsatellite markers by determining the average of the values for all possible allele combinations of the two markers weighted by the marginal allele probabilities.

8. Carry out single-point and haplotype association comparing the patient group with controls. Fisher-exact test is one way to test for single-point association. Haplotype association is quite challenging in most common diseases, as the parents are not available for most patients with late-onset disease. There are a variety of programs available for defining haplotypes and looking for disease association. Many derive haplotypes using an expectation maximization (EM) algorithm that uses LD to help define most likely haplotypes. Then the most likely haplotypes defined are tested for association with a Fisher exact test. However, the resulting *p* value of the difference does not take into account the uncertainty of defining the haplotypes tested; it may require randomization to properly

evaluate statistical significance. However, other programs such as NEsted MOdels (NEMO), developed at Decode, do attempt to account for the uncertainty in haplotype estimation when reporting the p value for association *(1,3)*. NEMO employs an extension of the EM algorithm. It was developed at Decode by Daniel Gudbjartsson and Augustine Kong *(3)*. Haplotype frequencies are estimated by maximum likelihood and the differences between patients and controls are tested using a generalized likelihood ratio test. The maximum likelihood estimates, likelihood ratios, and p values are computed with the aid of the EM algorithm directly for the observed data, and, hence, the loss of information owing to the uncertainty with phase and missing genotypes is automatically captured by the likelihood ratios, and under most situations, large-sample theory can be used to reliably determine statistical significance. In NEMO, a model is defined by a partition of the set of all possible haplotypes where haplotypes in the same group are assumed to confer the same risk whereas haplotypes in different groups can confer different risks. A null hypothesis and an alternative hypothesis are nested when the latter corresponds to a finer partition than the former. NEMO provides complete flexibility in the partition of the haplotype space. That allowed us, in work in which we discovered a gene conferring substantial risk for ischemic stroke *(3)*, to partition haplotypes into three groups—an at-risk group for stroke, a protective group and the wild-type group. NEMO can use the multiplicative, or haplotype relative risk, model, but it can also test haplotypes for correlation continuous traits.

9. Interpret the association results. Although there are no accepted criteria to define statistical significance of a haplotype or SNP association within a region first defined by a linkage peak, in general, we apply the following basic criteria internally:

   a. The haplotype or gene must show the most significant association (lowest p value defined carefully with an algorithm like NEMO to ensure that the uncertainty in definition of phase within the haplotype is accounted for) within the one-lod drop.

   b. The entire one-lod drop must be typed with sufficient number of markers to define the LD blocks in the region and ensure that there are no large marker-free gaps between LD blocks.

   c. The haplotype must replicate in a second independent Icelandic cohort or a cohort from another country.

   p values can be corrected for multiple testing of the markers conservatively by a Bonferoni correction (that is, multiplying the nominal p value by the number of independent tests). This is more straightforward to apply to the single-point association results. For haplotype association, the number of independent tests is not so clear. Alternatively and less conservatively, correction of the p value can be done by randomizing the patient and control groups and repeating the association numerous times to determine the number of times a give association is seen by chance. In practice, for a 6-Mb region containing 200–500 markers, our experience suggests that nominal p values for haplotype association would need to be in the range 10^{-5} to 10^{-6} to survive multiple testing corrections. Although this sounds very stringent, it is three orders of magnitude better than the *p* values needed from a genome-wide association study.

10. Although it appears that most low-penetrant variants contributing to common diseases are not missense or nonsense mutations, it is useful to carry out mutation screening of at least the exons and upstream promoter region to detect rare disease-associated variants.

11. Check for population stratification. Association studies should be run individually on ethnic subgroups and not mixed. However, to decrease the chance of false-positive association from differences due to population stratification, it will be important to confirm the self-reported ethnicity in each group and to ensure that the genetic backgrounds of the patient group match that of the control groups. Microsatellite marker sets are especially informative in distinguishing major ethnic groups. To evaluate genetically estimated ancestry of the study cohorts, we use a panel of 75 unlinked microsatellite markers from about 2000 microsatellites genotyped in a multi-ethnic cohort of 35 European Americans from Baltimore, 88 African-Americans from Pittsburgh, Baltimore, and North Carolina, 34 Chinese (Canton), and 29 Indian Americans (Zapotec. Of the 2000 microsatellite markers, the selected set showed the most significant differences between the European Americans, African Americans, and Asians, and implicitly Indians, and also had good quality and yield. Thirty-one of these markers were also used for similar purposes in a recent study by Tang et al. *(15)*.

Using genotype data from these markers on the ethnic plates, Structure software will estimate the genetic background of test individuals *(16,17)*. Structure infers the allele frequencies of K ancestral populations on the basis of multilocus genotypes from a set of individuals and a user-specified value of K, and assigns a proportion of ancestry from each of the inferred K populations to each individual. We can use the ethnicity panel in two ways. First, we include in the analysis only those Caucasians who have at least 90% European ancestry in patients and controls. Second, we have modified the NEMO haplotype association algorithm to adjust for differences in genetic background between cases and controls so that we can include all Caucasians according to self-report.

4. Notes

1. It is helpful (and essential in any moderate- or high-throughput genetics facility) to have a barcoding and tracking system that is tied to a comprehensive LIMS system. The system should be connected to a sample database that tracks blood tube and DNA tube storage along with their respective histories of intake, conversion, transfer, and use.

2. The data generated from each marker are scrutinized for genotyping yield, mismatches with previous determinations of the same marker-person combination, and deviations from Hardy-Weinberg equilibrium. Genotypes that pass these QC

steps are lifted into a high quality database by a proprietary "bucket-wheel" software mechanism called the QC-Demon. If subsequent genotyping data relating to a marker or marker-person combination shows a problem, the QC-Demon removes all discordant genotypes from the high quality database. Inheritance error checks are used to monitor marker performance and to detect misidentified DNA samples. Relationship checks operate at a more global level to check the integrity of the pedigrees. The relationship between each pair of first- or second-degree relatives is checked by comparing the identity-by-state (IBS) of their entire framework microsatellite set genotypes to the expected IBS for the relationship generated from a training sample using the same marker set. Incorrect relationships are corrected in accordance to these results. If the relationship cannot be resolved, then the uncertain connection is severed.

3. Power of an association study. Number of patients and controls required to have 80 or 90% power to detect an association with a two-sided p value of 10^{-5} for various risk ratios and population frequency of an allele/haplotype.

Frequency of haplotype in Controls	RR = 1.5		RR = 2.0		RR = 3.0	
	80%	90%	80%	90%	80%	90%
0.05	2951	3465	888	1043	296	348
0.10	1594	2204	490	576	170	199
0.15	1152	1352	356	424	129	152
0.20	939	1102	300	352	111	130
0.25	819	962	266	313	101	118
0.30	747	877	247	290	96	113

4. Microsatellite markers found using the tandem repeat finder (TRF) program *(18)* Primers are designed using adequate criteria for PCR assays, and primers that include repeats or known SNPs in the sequence are excluded. The likelihood of a successful microsatellite, that is, a readable and polymorphic marker, is estimated by associating the characteristics of the microsatellite, including monomer length, microsatellite length, and repeat structure, with experimental success in a set of over 25,000 microsatellite markers previously designed and tested at DECODE. We use this to rank the putative microsatellites according to expected quality, and we have identified more than 40,000 putative microsatellites in the genome that we classify as rank 1. In our experience, more than 70% of these turn out to be usable.

5. It is important to encrypt all personal identifiers before they arrive in the laboratory. All personal identifiers are reversibly coded by the Data Protection Commission outside our laboratory to prevent identification of any particular individual *(19)*.

References

1. Helgadottir, A., Manolescu, A., Thorleifsson, G., et al. (2004) The gene encoding 5-lipoxygenase activating protein confers risk of myocardial infarction and stroke. *Nat. Genet.* **36**, 233–239.

2. Helgadottir, A., Gretarsdottir, S., St. Clair, D., et al. (2005) Association between the gene encoding 5-Lipoxygenase-activating protein and stroke replicated in a scottish population. *Am. J. Hum. Genet.* **76,** 505–509.
3. Gretarsdottir, S., Thorleifsson, G., Reynisdottir, S. T., et al. (2003) The gene encoding Phosphodiesterase 4D confers risk of ischemic stroke. *Nat. Genet.* **35,** 131–138.
4. Gudmundsson, G., Matthiasson, S. E., Arason, H., et al.(2002) Localization of a gene for peripheral arterial occlusive disease to chromosome 1p31. *Am. J. Hum. Genet.* **70,** 586–592.
5. Polak, R. A., et al. (1999) Carotid-artery intima and media thickness as a risk factor for myocardial infarction and stroke in older adults. Cardiovascular Health Study Collaborative Research Group. *N. Engl. J. Med .* **340,** 14–22.
6. Fox, C. S., Polak J. F., Chazaro I., et al. (2003) Genetic and environmental contributions to atherosclerosis phenotypes in men and women: heritability of carotid intima-media thickness in the Framingham Heart Study. *Stroke* **34,** 397–401.
7. Kong, A., Gudbjartsson, D. F., Sainz, J., et al. (2002) A high-resolution recombination map of the human genome. *Nat. Genet.* **31,** 241–247.
8. Gudbjartsson, D. F., Jonasson, K., Frigge, M. L., and Kong, A. (2000) Allegro, a new computer program for multipoint linkage analysis. *Nat. Genet.* **25,** 12–13.
9. Kong, A. and Cox, N. J. (1997) Allele-sharing models: LOD scores and accurate linkage tests. *Am. J. Hum. Genet.* **61,** 1179–1188.
10. Kruglyak, L., Daly, M. J., Reeve-Daly, M. P., and Lander, E. S. (1996) Parametric and nonparametric linkage analysis: a unified multipoint approach. *Am. J. Hum. Genet.* **58,** 1347–1363.
11. Nicolae, D. L. (1999) Allele sharing models in gene mapping: a likelihood approach. PhD Thesis, Department of Statistics, University of Chicago, Chicago, IL: pp. 126.
12. Dempster, A. P., Laird, N. M., and Rubin, D. B. (1977) Maximum likelihood estimation from incomplete data via the EM algorithm (with discussion). *J. R. Stat. Soc. Ser. B Stat. Med.* **39,** 1–38.
13. Lander, E. and Kruglyak, L. (1995) Genetic dissection of complex traits: guidelines for interpreting and reporting linkage results. *Nat. Genet.* **11,** 241–247.
14. Stefansson, H., Sigurdsson, E., Steinthorsdottir, V., et al. (2002). Neuregulin 1 and susceptibility to schizophrenia. *Am. J. Hum. Genet.* **71,** 877–892.
15. Tang, H., Quertermous, T., Rodriguez, B., et al. (2005) Genetic structure, self-identified race/ethnicity, and confounding in case-control association studies. *Am. J. Hum. Genet.* **76,** 268–275.
16. Falush, D., Stephens, M., and Pritchard, J. K. (2003) Inference of population structure using multilocus genotype data: linked loci and correlated allele frequencies. *Genetics* **164,** 1567–1587.
17. Pritchard, J. K., Stephens, M., and Donnelly, P. (2000) Inference of population structure using multilocus genotype data. *Genetics* **155,** 945–959.
18. Benson, G. (1999). Tandem repeats finder: a program to analyze DNA sequences. *Nucleic Acids Res.* **27,** 573–580.

19. Gulcher, J. R., Kristjansson, K., Gudbjartsson, H., and Stefansson, K. (2000) Protection of privacy by third-party encryption in genetic research in Iceland. *Eur. J. Hum. Genet* **8,** 739–742.

11

Chromosome Substitution Strains

A New Way to Study Genetically Complex Traits

Annie E. Hill, Eric S. Lander, and Joseph H. Nadeau

Summary

Many biological traits and heritable diseases are multifactorial, involving combinations of genetic variants and environmental factors. To dissect the genetic basis for these traits and to characterize their functional consequences, mouse models are widely used, not only because of their genetic and physiological similarity to humans, but also because an extraordinary variety of genetic resources enable rigorous functional studies. Chromosome substitution strains (CSSs) are a powerful complement to existing resources for studying multigenic traits. By partitioning the genome into a panel of new inbred strains with single chromosome substitutions, one strain for each of the autosomes, the X and Y chromosome, and the mitochondria, unique experimental designs and considerable statistical power are possible. Multigenic trait genes (or quantitative trait loci [QTLs]) with weak effects are easily detected, linkage and congenic crosses can be quickly made, gene interactions are readily characterized, and discovery of QTLs is greatly accelerated. Several published studies demonstrate the considerable utility of these strains and new applications for CSSs continue to be discovered.

Key Words: Chromosome substitution strains; congenic strains; complex traits; quantitative trait loci; QTLs; linkage crosses; epistasis.

1. The Genetics of Complex Traits

Understanding the complexities of phenotypic variation in health and dysfunction is important to satisfy our curiosity about the natural world and to discover ways to diagnose and treat disease. Many genes, acting alone and in combination, influence most traits and diverse environmental factors modulate their actions. Even simple Mendelian traits show evidence of complex influences through the action of modifier genes *(1)*. By identifying these various genes, characterizing their interactions and defining their biological functions, we will learn about the manner in which genetic codes are translated into

From: *Methods in Molecular Medicine, Vol. 128: Cardiovascular Disease; Methods and Protocols; Volume 1*
Edited by: Q. Wang © Humana Press Inc., Totowa, NJ

organismal forms and functions. We can also discover the ways in which functionality is maintained despite genetic and environmental perturbations, which is key to studies of systems biology.

Finding the genes that control phenotypic variation and that cause disease is challenging. With genome sequences and single-nucleotide polymorphism (SNP) maps, the locations and nature of sequence variants that code for functional diversity are being rapidly cataloged (2–9). Powerful and sensitive ways to engineer mice with specific sequence variants and with controlled gene expression patterns are being developed. The rate-limiting step is obtaining sufficient recombination events in planned crosses and in existing stocks, families, and populations. Various strategies are being used to map genes based on high-resolution mapping crosses and linkage disequilibrium in association tests. These crossovers identify the short list of candidate sequence variants for functional testing.

Quantitative trait loci (QTLs) are being identified at an increasing rate in humans, mice, and other species, both in linkage and in association studies (10–14) Some of these are conventional QTLs and others are modifier genes. These genes and their sequence variants provide clues to the control of biological processes in health and disease.

But progress in gene discovery remains slow. For most traits, the combined action of known QTLs fails to account for the majority of the genetic variation in trait differences; finding ways to detect more trait-controlling genes is critical so that a complete catalog of genes is available for functional studies. More efficient ways to make congenic strains and other specially engineered strains and crosses are needed. Typically, these take years to make. The extent to which gene interactions complicate the detection, mapping, and identification of complex trait genes remains to be determined; new and powerful ways to detect and characterize these interactions are urgently needed.

Many genetic strategies are being used to find QTLs. These include segregating crosses, recombinant inbred strains, recombinant congenic strains, advanced inbred strains, heterogeneous stocks, and other unique genetic resources (15–19). These are invariably based on the principle of random genetic segregation, either with crosses or with inbred strains in which recombinant chromosomes have been homozygosed. In this paradigm, depending on the analytical methods used, each genetic point or interval is tested to determine whether a genetic variant at that locus contributes significantly to phenotypic variation. Each test determines whether individuals of alternative genotypes at a given locus (or interval) differ significantly given the genetic heterogeneity of the study population. Because all of the trait-controlling genetic variants in the genome segregate simultaneously, the challenge is detecting the signal of each QTL against the background "noise" of all other segregating QTLs.

Chromosome substitution strains (CSSs) are based on a different paradigm that deal with the signal–noise problem in a novel way *(20)*. Each CSSs is an inbred strain that differs from the host strain by a single intact and homozygous chromosome on a defined and uniform genetic background. In a CSS panel, the genome is partitioned into a series of strains in which each chromosome is substituted onto the host inbred background. As a result, each chromosome, i.e., each CSS, can be interrogated independently for QTLs that affect the trait of interest while the action of QTLs on all other chromosomes is held constant. This strategy reduces the "noise" of other QTLs and consequently leads to a dramatic improvement in the signal-to-noise ratio.

In this chapter, we review the construction of CSSs, their applications, several statistical and analytical issues, and selected results from recent studies.

2. General Principles

We describe here the general principles for making and analyzing CSSs; detailed logistics to make, use, and analyze CSSs are described in subsequent sections. CSSs are made with methods that are similar to those used to make congenic strains (**Fig. 1**). The first step is to select a host and donor strain. The second step is to transfer each chromosome from the donor strain to the host strain with repeated backcrosses and selection for mice that inherit the nonrecombinant chromosome of interest at each backcross generation. The third step is to homozygose the substituted chromosome. With a complete panel of CSSs, a genome survey is simple—the trait is measured in each CSS and trait results compared for each CSS to the host strain. A significant difference demonstrates that at least one QTL is located on that substituted chromosome.

3. Detecting QTLs

The first, and often neglected, problem in complex trait analysis is QTL detection. Many QTLs are thought to control complex traits. But in most studies relatively few are detected *(10–14)*. Conventional approaches are, therefore, appropriate for sampling the variety of genes that contribute to complex traits. But in many kinds of studies, especially studies of systems biology, a more complete QTL catalogue is needed for modeling and functional analyses.

A key problem is detecting the signal for each QTL against the phenotypic "noise" of all other segregating QTLs. With adequate statistical power, QTLs with strong effects are readily detected, but those with weak effects elude detection. Effect size is a useful measure of the contribution of a QTL to total genetic variation. It is measured as the fractional contribution (typically in expressed as a percentage) of each detected QTL to the overall difference in trait means between the parental strains. Detected QTLs usually have an effect size of 3–7% *(13,14)*. Statistical considerations suggest that ability to detect

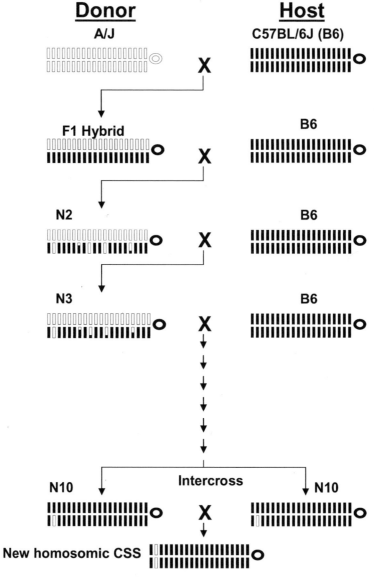

Donor

Host

Fig. 1. Substituting chromosomes. In this example, the A/J inbred donor strain is crossed to the C57BL/6J (B6) inbred host strain to produce F1 hybrids. These hybrids are backcrossed to the B6 host strain to produce N2 heterozygous progeny which are genotyped for the chromosome of interest, in this case chromosome 2. N2 mice that inherited a nonrecombinant version of chromosome 2 from the A/J donor strain are backcrossed to the B6 host strain to produce N3 progeny in which the mice are again genotyped for nonrecombinant A/J for chromosome 2. This process of backcrossing and genotypic selection is repeated at each backcross generation to N10. Heterosomic

QTLs declines rapidly as their effect size becomes smaller—an expectation that is supported by considerable empirical evidence *(13,14)*. The typical solution is to increase statistical power with more markers and especially larger sample sizes.

The use of a CSS panel to map QTLs is simple. The trait value for each QTL is compared to the host strain and significant differences implicate at least one QTL on the substituted chromosome. Although the number of QTLs and their locations is uncertain, the implicated CSS can be used to address both questions (*see* **Subheading 4.**). For CSSs that do not differ significantly from the host strain, several interpretations are possible. First, there may not be QTLs on that substituted chromosome. Second, the QTLs may have relatively weak effects and eluded detection because of sample size and statistical power. Third, the substituted chromosome may have several QTLs that act in contrasting directions to increase or alternatively to reduce the trait value, so that the trait means for the CSS and the host strain do not differ significantly.

An important advantage of CSSs is that subsequent genetic and functional studies are readily pursued after a CSS is identified. For example, congenic strains are readily made from the CSS, mapping crosses can be made with the CSS, and functional studies are immediately possible with the CSSs as well as the strains and crosses derived from them.

4. Mapping QTLs

4.1. CSS Crosses

Two kinds of intercrosses and backcrosses can be made with CSSs. The first kind is used to determine the number and location of QTLs on the substituted chromosome, and the alternative kind cross-fixes the QTL on the substituted chromosome and studies the action of QTLs on all other chromosomes. For the former, which focus on the genetics of the substituted chromosome, crosses are made between the CSS of interest and the host strain (**Fig. 2A**). The resulting hybrids can then be intercrossed or alternatively they can be backcrossed to either parental strain. Regardless of the nature or direction of these crosses, the segregating genome is confined to the substituted chromosome; the remainder of the genome is identical for the host strain and the CSS. Restricting segregation to a single chromosome has many statistical and analytical advantages (*see* **Subheading 6.**). Because several unique attributes of CSSs provide important statistical advantages, comparatively small samples are needed to

---

Fig. 1. *(continued from opposite page)* mice are intercrossed and genotyped to identify homosomic progeny. In addition, special considerations are needed to the substitutions to ensure that the X and Y chromosomes as well as the mitochondria are derived from the host or donor strains, as appropriate (*see* **Subheadings 5.1.2.2.–5.1.2.4.**).

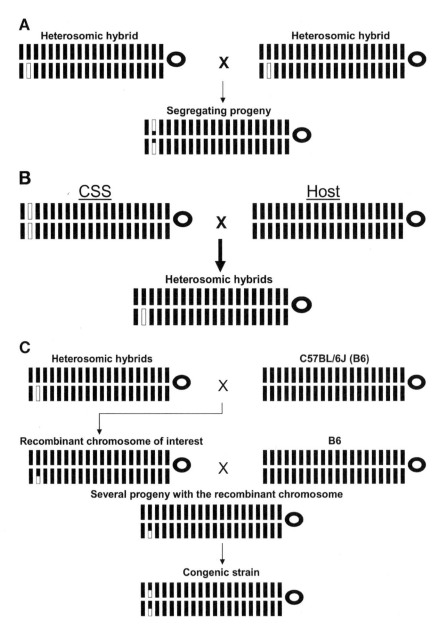

Fig. 2. (**A**) Linkage tests with chromosome substitution strain (CSS) intercrosses. Hybrids are intercrossed and progeny are phenotyped and genotyped as in standard intercrosses, except the segregating "genome" is a single chromosome. (**B**) Tests for dominance. By crossing a CSS to its host strain, for example, B6.Chr2$^{A/J}$ (CSS) × C57BL/6J, only the chromosome that is substituted is heterosomic while the background is homosomic for the host genome, thereby enabling a direct test of dominance

determine the number and location of QTLs on the substituted chromosome. The progeny can then be genotyped (with various kinds of genetic markers that span the length of the substituted chromosome) and phenotyped (with assays relevant to the trait of interest).

With respect to the latter kind of crosses, which focus on the genetics of residual effects, the CSS of interest is crossed to the donor strain and the resulting hybrids can be intercrossed or backcrossed to the CSS or to the donor strain. In these crosses, the action of QTLs on the substituted chromosome is fixed and segregation of QTLs in the remainder of the genome can be studied. This strategy can be helpful in many studies, but especially when the effect of a strong QTL masks the action of other QTLs.

4.2. Tests for Dominance Effects

In many studies, it is important to determine whether the traits are inherited in a dominant (or recessive) manner. (It is important to remember that dominance is a property of an individual, rather than a specific allele, and therefore it depends on the genetic constitution of the individual or strain being studied.) CSSs can be used to dissect the genetic control of dominance. By crossing the CSS with the host strain, dominance effects can be assessed (**Fig. 2B**).

4.3. Congenic Strains

Congenic strains are an indispensable resource in many genetic and functional studies *(15,21)*. Typically, a congenic strain is made with at least 10 backcross generations to the host strain and selection at each backcross for mice with the trait or chromosome segment of interest. Making a congenic strain requires 2–3 yr. The process can be accelerated by conducting genome scans on progeny at each backcross generation *(22)*. These "speed congenics" accelerate production of the strain at a cost of genotyping large numbers of mice.

CSSs uniquely speed production of congenic strains, because the background is already isogenic with the host strain (**Fig. 2C**). Hybrids resulting from crosses between the CSS and the host strain are backcrossed to the host strain. Progeny are genotyped with genetic markers to identify progeny that inherit relevant recombinant chromosomes. These mice are selected for another backcross to the host strain and progeny with the recombinant chromosome of interest are then intercrossed to homozygose the chromosome. This process requires as few as four crosses and can be completed in less than 1 yr and with

---

Fig. 2. *(continued from opposite page)* without complicating background effects. (**C**) Congenic strains from CSSs. Standard methods for making a congenic strain are used *(15,21)*, except that the starting material is a CSS rather than a conventional inbred strain.

limited genotyping. With individual congenic strains or with a complete panel of congenic strain that partition the chromosome into a series of overlapping segments, conventional methods of congenic strain analysis can be used for QTL mapping and functional studies.

5. Making CSSs

To construct the B6-Chr$^{A/J}$ CSS panel, we selected two inbred strains, with C57BL/6J (B6) as the host strain and A/J as the donor strain. These strains, like most other strains, differ in an extraordinary variety of traits from transcription levels to life-span, from molecules such as amino acids and lipids to organs such as heart and kidney, and from innate traits to induced traits (*23–25*; www.jax.org/phenome). As a result, interesting traits can be studied in most strain combinations.

An equally important consideration is the compatibility of progenitor genomes. Although each inbred strain is homozygous for a combination of alleles that provide adequate viability and fertility to maintain the strain and appropriate behaviors to interact with cage-mates and researchers, mixing genomes of different inbred strains often yields allelic combinations that compromise the new inbred strains. Success with mixed genomes varies dramatically among strain combinations. In our case, several of the largest panels of recombinant inbred and recombinant congenic strains were made with A/J and B6 as progenitors (*21*). We were therefore confident that these genomes were reasonably compatible with each other and that a complete panel of CSSs could be made with the A/J and B6 strains.

Making a CSS, or a panel of CSSs, requires several logistical considerations. Each CSS must have a single substituted chromosome from the donor strain while assuring that all other chromosomes are derived from the host strain. Simple backcrosses, without regard to the "direction" of the cross, are adequate to ensure that autosomes are transferred. However, the gender of the mice, and, hence, the "direction" of the cross, is important to ensure that the X and Y chromosomes and the mitochondria are derived from the host strain in autosomal CSSs. In the following sections, we describe in detail the steps required to transfer each autosome, each of the sex chromosomes, and the mitochondria. We also describe the genotyping methods to identify nonrecombinant chromosomes and the frequencies of heterosomic and homosomic mice in the various crosses.

5.1. Steps for Making a CSS

5.1.1. Selecting the Host and Donor Strains

In addition to the biological and compatibility issues, there is another factor to consider before making CSSs: existing CSSs may be appropriate for the planned studies. In our experience, and that of many of our collaborators, phenotypes vary considerable among inbred strains. The prototypic strains for particular traits are sometime accidents of discovery, and other strain combinations may be as informative. The Mouse Phenome Project shows that most traits vary among many inbred strains (*23–25; see also* www.jax.org/phenome). Researchers are therefore encouraged to test progenitors to determine whether existing CSSs might be useful.

5.1.2. Crosses to Substitute Autosomes From the Donor Strain

5.1.2.1. CROSSES

At each backcross generation, mice are surveyed to identify those that inherit a nonrecombinant chromosome that is derived from the donor strain. Mice with nonrecombinant chromosomes are crossed to the host strain for at least 10 consecutive backcross generations if Marker-Assisted Selection (MAS; *see* **Subheading 5.1.7.**) is not used, and for fewer generations if MAS is used. After the appropriate number of backcrosses, heterosomic mice are then intercrossed to obtain homosomic progeny, which are brother–sister mated to maintain each CSS. Although this is the general approach, we also used several minor but important modifications to improve efficiency.

5.1.2.2. ENSURING THAT IN AUTOSOMAL CSSs THE Y CHROMOSOME IS DERIVED FROM THE HOST STRAIN

In at least one backcross, females from the donor strain, or alternatively, heterosomic females, are crossed to males from the host strain. With these females, the Y chromosome from the donor strain is lost from the incipient CSS; in all subsequent crosses, both male and female progeny can be used because the Y chromosome is obligately derived from the host strain.

Exemplar: *Crosses at the first generation, where d = donor and h = host.*
$X_d X_d$ donor females $\times$ $X_h Y_h$ host males yields $X_d Y_h$ F1 males,
then, $X_h X_h$ host females $\times$ $X_d Y_h$ F1 males yields $X_h Y_h$ F1 males.

Exemplar: *Crosses at later backcross generations where i = d, h or recombinant.*
$X_i X_i$ incipient CSS females $\times$ $X_h Y_h$ host males yields $X_i Y_h$ males
then, $X_h X_h$ host females $\times$ $X_i Y_h$ incipient CSS males yields $X_h Y_h$ F1 females.

5.1.2.3. ENSURING THAT IN AUTOSOMAL CSSs THE X CHROMOSOME IS DERIVED FROM THE HOST STRAIN

To make certain that each autosomal CSS has the X chromosome from the host strain, females from the host strain are crossed to males from the donor strain, in the first-generation crosses. Hybrid males are then crossed to host strain females:

Exemplar: crosses at the first generation.
X_hX_h host females $\quad\quad\quad\times\quad X_dY_d$ donor males yields X_hY_d F1 hybrid males,
then, X_hX_h host females $\quad\times\quad X_hY_d$ F1 hybrid males yields X_hX_h females.

Exemplar: crosses at later backcross generations.
X_hX_i incipient CSS females $\times\quad _hY_h$ host male $\quad\quad\quad$ yields X_hX_h incipient
CSS females and X_hY_h
incipient CSS males,
then, X_hX_h incipient $\quad\quad\times\quad X_hY_h$ host males $\quad\quad$ yields X_hY_h incipient
CSS females CSS males,
or X_hY_h incipient $\quad\quad\quad\times\quad X_hX_h$ host females $\quad$ yields X_hX_h incipient
CSS males CSS females.

5.1.2.4. KEEPING THE MITOCHONDRIA FROM THE HOST STRAIN

Mitochondria are inherited through the maternal lineage, with rare exception. Thus, deriving the incipient CSS from progeny of females from the host strain, for at least one generation, is sufficient to make certain that the mitochondria are derived thereafter from the host strain.

5.1.2.5. SEQUENCE OF STEPS

In general, several sequences are possible. Once a chromosome has been fixed, it cannot be lost as long as attention is paid to the nature and direction of the crosses and the sequence of steps.

5.1.3. Substituting the Chromosome X From the Donor Strain

Females from the donor strain are crossed to males from the host strain and at each generation male and female progeny are tracked to follow inheritance of the X_d chromosome. Progeny of hemisomic X_dY_i males do not need to be genotyped because the X chromosome does not recombine in males (except for the pseudoautosomal region). By contrast, progeny of heterosomic X_dX_i females must be genotyped. With the appropriate arrangement of crosses, genotyping is therefore required only in alternate generations.

5.1.4. Substituting the Chromosome Y From the Donor Strain

Males from the donor strain are crossed to females from the host strain at the first generation, and then male progeny are used in crosses to host strain females in each subsequent backcross generation. After at least 10 backcross generations, additional backcrosses can be used to maintain the strain (recommended) or brother–sister matings can be used. DNA-based genotyping is not required.

5.1.5. Substituting Mitochondria From the Donor Strain

Females from the donor strain are crossed to males from the host strain at the first generation and then female progeny are used at each subsequent backcross to the host strain. After 10 backcross generations, either additional back-crosses or brother–sister matings can be used.

5.1.6. Genotyping: Identifying Mice With Nonrecombinant Chromosomes

At each backcross generation, mice with a nonrecombinant chromosome are identified by typing a panel of markers that span the chromosome from telom-ere to telomere. The markers can be simple sequence length polymorphisms (SSLPs), SNPs, or other appropriate markers that distinguish one chromosome from the other. Several markers should be as close to the ends of the chromo-some as possible to make certain that the ends of the chromosome are not lost because of undetected crossovers. Additional markers that are located between the flanking markers can be used to identify mice with double-crossovers. These markers guard against crossovers that would compromise the integrity of the chromosome. The number of these intervening markers is somewhat arbitrary because small double-crossovers are rare.

The frequency of mice that inherit a nonrecombinant chromosome is critical to the success of making CSSs. Based on a sample of more than 17,000 mice that were genotyped during construction of the B6-Chr$^{A/J}$ panel, the frequency of mice with a nonrecombinant chromosome is approx 40% and of that, half (~20% of the total number of progeny) were heterosomic for the nonrecom-binant chromosome of interest *(26)*. Thus, in a litter of five, on average one will have the appropriate nonrecombinant chromosome.

As expected, most recombinant chromosomes had a single crossover, and chromosomes with more than one crossover were rare. These are expected to be uncommon simply based on statistical considerations. However, they are less frequent than expected because of interference *(27)*. For poorly under-stood reasons, occurrence of a single crossover inhibits additional crossovers. An important implication of strong interference is that the number of markers that are needed to survey chromosomes is greatly reduced.

5.1.7. Speed-Consomics With Marker-Assisted Selection

The original purpose of marker-assisted selection (MAS) is to accelerate production of congenic strains by identifying backcross progeny that by chance inherited more of the host strain background than other segregants *(22)*. By selectively breeding these, the rate of loss of chromosome segments that are derived from the donor strain can be accelerated. To find these optimal seg-regants, large numbers of backcross progeny are typed for genetic markers throughout the genome. Obviously, the chance of finding an optimal segregant increases with larger numbers of surveyed backcross progeny.

Several logistical issues should be considered. First, without MAS, 50% of the donor genome will be lost at each generation. The benefits of MAS are therefore an incremental benefit over these simple Mendelian advantages. The major cost in this approach is the number of backcross mice that are surveyed at each generation, with greater numbers leading a greater chance of obtaining the appropriate segregant. So the "price" to accelerate the backcrossing is increased numbers of both markers and mice to genotype at each generation. With increasing availability of readily typed genetic markers and with the rapidly improving genotyping technologies, the feasibility of MAS improves dramatically. Using MAS to make a CSS is a simple extension of these principles.

5.1.8. Homozygosing the Selected Chromosome

In our experience, this is the most challenging step because homosomic mice are rare among progeny of heterosomic intercrosses. In general, with a 20% frequency of heterosomic mice, the frequency of homosomic mice is only approx 4%, simply because transmission of the nonrecombinant chromosome from *both* parents is needed. Again, the rate depends in part on the genetic length of the selected chromosome, with lower rates occurring for longer chromosomes.

To make the B6-Chr$^{A/J}$ panel of CSSs, we modified the design of the crosses to accommodate these low rates. When a homosomic mouse was found among progeny of heterosomic intercrosses, it was crossed to a heterosomic mouse. In these crosses, 20% of the progeny were homosomic. Thus, a reasonable number of homosomic mice could be collected in a short time. From these, homosomic crosses were made to establish the CSSs.

5.1.9. Genome Scans to Verify CSS Integrity

It is essential to verify the integrity of the substituted chromosomes to make certain that they are intact that they do not have undetected double-crossovers. Equally important is a survey to make certain that unselected chromosome segments do not accidentally persist from the donor strain. In principle, 10 backcross generations is sufficient to lose all unselected chromosome segments from the donor strain. Sometimes, however, unselected segments of other chromosomes persist either by chance or because of functional interactions with the selected chromosome. A genome survey can reveal these segments and additional crosses used to remove the unwanted content from the CSS. An important consideration is the density of markers to be used for these genome surveys. Obviously, high-density surveys have a greater ability to detect small chromosome segments. As genotyping methods improve and costs decline, higher density surveys will become possible. An important advantage of CSSs is that if a problem is discovered or a strain lost, a new CSS is readily made again. Other resources such as recombinant inbred strains are genetically unique and can not be replicated.

6. Statistical and Analytical Issues

Multiple testing penalties arise in every genome survey. In general, these can be resolved with the guidelines proposed by Lander and Kruglyak *(28)* or with permutation tests *(29)*. In either case, the penalties are substantial and as a result the power of most studies is greatly limited. The typical solution is to increase the sample size substantially. CSSs resolve this problem in a unique way with important implications.

Because a genome survey simply involves testing each CSS one at a time, the number of tests is simply the haploid number of chromosomes in the genome plus 2 (to account for the two sex chromosomes and the mitochondria). Moreover, because each CSS is genetically distinct from all others in the panel, the complete genome survey for mice involves *independent* comparisons only, one for each of the autosomes, one each for the X and Y chromosomes, and one for the mitochondria. For the mouse, N + 2 = 22. As a result, simple Bonferroni corrections are adequate to account for multiple testing *(26,30)*.

An important consequence of linkage testing crosses with CSSs is that the segregating genome is a single chromosome rather than the entire genome. As a result, the penalties for multiple testing in CSS mapping crosses are reduced dramatically. The Lander-Kruglyak methods are readily modified by using the genetic length of the substituted chromosome rather than the total genetic length of the genome.

In general, the threshold required to declare significant evidence for linkage is reduced 30-fold and to declare suggestive evidence for linkage is reduced 20-fold *(30)*. If a single QTL controls the trait of interest, the sample size needed to declare linkage is 37% smaller than with conventional crosses. This advantage increases with increasing genetic complexity *(26)*. Finally, heritability of traits tends to be approximately threefold higher in CSSs than in conventional crosses *(30)*. Together, these attributes make CSSs a statistically robust platform for QTL detection and mapping.

7. History of CSSs

In the early days of genetics, construction of CSSs depended on various genetic "tricks" to avoid recombination. CSSs, which were pioneered in fly and plant genetics, have been used to study body weight in flies and many quantitative traits in wheat *(31–35)*. In many cases, heterozygosity for chromosome inversions, which suppresses crossing-over, was used to ensure transfer of intact nonrecombinant chromosomes from the donor strain to the host strain.

In mice, several CSSs involving the Y chromosome were constructed to study various sex-limited traits *(20)*. These CSSs were readily made simply by using males at each backcross generation because the Y chromosome does not recombine—except for its pseudoautosomal portion, which recombines regularly with the corresponding portion of the X chromosome.

Availability of readily typed genetic markers revolutionized construction of CSSs by enabling identification of nonrecombinant chromosomes in segregating crosses (20). The first autosomal CSS was made with SSLPs as genetic markers (36). Recently, Singer et al. reported the first complete panel of CSSs (all chromosomes) (26). Completing this panel required more than 17,000 SSLP-genotyped mice and more than 7 yr. Advances in genotyping technologies, namely SNP maps, make it feasible to complete a CSS panel in perhaps as few as 4 yr.

8. Studies With CSSs

8.1. Detecting QTLs

Relatively few of the many genes that control complex traits are detected with conventional analytical methods. The detected QTLs typically explain a modest fraction of the total genetic variation. Moreover, without a map location for the undetected QTLs, most genetic studies are compromised. The first challenge is therefore detecting as many QTLs as possible in part to characterize the genetic architecture of biological and disease traits and in part to increase the number of proteins that might be used as drug targets. Because of the unique manner in which CSSs enhance the signal-to-noise ratio, CSSs offer the possibility of detecting more QTLs and therefore accounting for more of the genetic variation. To illustrate the power of CSSs, we compared the numbers of QTLs detected with conventional methods and with CSSs (26). For traits such as obesity, cholesterol and sitosterol, conventional methods detect 1–4 QTLs, whereas CSSs detect 8–20 QTLs (**Fig. 3**). Thus, significantly more QTLs are routinely detected in CSS surveys than in conventional crosses.

8.2. Testicular Cancer

Testicular cancer is a polygenic threshold trait (36–38). Few susceptibility genes have been mapped and none have been identified. Conventional linkage crosses have to date failed to detect even suggestive evidence for linkage. A survey of more than 11,000 intercross and backcross progeny revealed a single affected mouse. This extraordinary level of genetic complexity precludes conventional methods for complex trait analysis. However, a linkage cross that was sensitized with a single-gene susceptibility mutation (*Ter*) revealed an appreciable frequency of affected mice (38). Sensitizing genetic studies with single-gene mutations has been used effectively in mutagenesis surveys, but has been largely neglected in complex trait analysis (39).

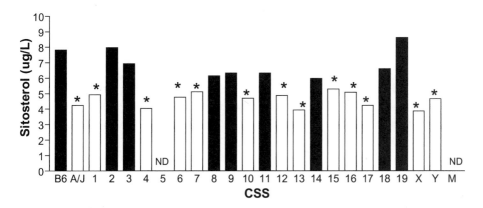

Fig. 3. Genetics of sitosterol levels in B6-Chr$_{A/J}$ CSSs. Thirteen of the 20 chromosome substitution strains (CSSs) have at least one quantitative trait locus affecting CSS levels (cf. **ref. 26**). Methods for measuring sitosterol levels are provided in reference 25. *Indicates a statistically significant difference between each CSS and the B6 host strain, after correction for multiple testing; ND indicates not done.

Instead of collecting more intercross progeny, with the hope of obtaining sufficient power to detect linkage, we constructed the first autosomal CSS— 129-Chr19^{MOLF} *(36)*. The best test score for linkage in several hundred segregating progeny did not reach the suggestive level of significance *(38)*. By contrast, the score in less than 30 CSS males was highly significant *(36)*, confirming the first linkage for a susceptibility gene for testicular cancer. The most likely location for this gene was near the center of the chromosome 19 linkage map. But the likelihood curve was broad, raising the possibility that several susceptibility genes are located on the substituted chromosome. A panel of single and double congenic strains was constructed *(37)*. We discovered that at least five enhancer and suppressor susceptibility genes act in additive or epistatic manners depending on the genetic composition of the chromosome. These congenic strains are now being used to identify the susceptibility genes and to characterize their effects on tumorigenesis. Without sensitized crosses and chromosome substitution strain, it is difficult to imagine that similar progress would have been made with conventional approaches.

8.3. Other Studies With CSSs

CSSs are being used to study the genetic control of an extraordinary variety of traits including resistance to testicular cancer *(36,37)*, γ-radiation-induced thymic lymphoma *(40)*, reproductive breakdown in hybrids between different subspecies *(41)*, prepulse inhibition *(42)*, airway hyper-responsiveness *(43)*, sex determination *(44)*, anxiety *(45)*, pubertal timing *(46)*, and mammary tumor progression and metastasis *(47)*.

9. CSS Resources

A complete panel of CSSs and several CSSs for other strain combinations are available (**Table 1**). Congenic strains have also been derived from several CSSs (**Table 2**). Other strains and panels are being developed, including the remainder of the A/J-Chr^{B6}, B6-Chr^{129} and 129-Chr^{B6} CSSs.

Finally, a panel of rat CSSs has been developed *(48)* and is being used to study a variety of physiological and molecular traits *(49,50)*.

10. Conclusion

The rich diversity of resources contributes to making the laboratory mouse an exceptional model for studying genetically complex traits. These resources include hundreds of inbred strains, recombinant inbred strains, recombinant congenic strains, advanced intercrosses and heterogeneous stocks, each of which has advantages and limitations *(9,14)*. By strategically selecting the right combination of genetic resources and mapping paradigms, it should be possible to quickly identify QTLs and to engineer new strains with special combinations of phenotypes. CSSs and congenic strains derived from them are ideal for detecting QTLs, for conducting detailed functional studies, and for phenotype engineering, whereas resources such as heterogeneous stocks are ideal for fine-mapping. Together, these resources are the foundation to address fundamental questions about the genetic basis of complex traits.

References

1. Nadeau, J. H. (2001) Modifier genes in mice and humans. *Nat. Rev. Genet.* **2,** 165–174.
2. Lindblad-Toh, K., Winchester, E., Daly, M. J., et al. (2000) Large-scale discovery and genotyping of single-nucleotide polymorphisms in the mouse. *Nat. Genet.* **24,** 381–386.
3. Wade, C. M., Kulbokas, E. J., Kirby, A. W., et al. (2002) The mosaic structure of variation in the laboratory mouse genome. *Nature* **420,** 574–578.
4. Wiltshire, T., Pletcher, M. T., Batalov, S., et al. (2003) Genome-wide single-nucleotide polymorphism analysis defines haplotype patterns in mouse. *Proc. Natl. Acad. Sci. USA* **100,** 3380–3385.
5. Ideraabdullah, F. Y., de la Casa-Esperon, E., Bell, T. A., et al. (2004) Genetic and haplotype diversity among wild-derived mouse inbred strains. *Genome Res.* **14,** 1880–1887.
6. Yalcin, B., Fullerton, J., Miller, S., et al. (2004) Unexpected complexity in the haplotypes of commonly used inbred strains of laboratory mice. *Proc. Natl. Acad. Sci. USA* **101,** 9734–9739.

Table 1
Available Chromosome Substitution Strains (CSSs): Host Strain, Donor Strain, Chomosome, and Contact

CSSs	Host	Donor	Chomosomes	Contact
C57BL/6J-Chr$^{A/J}$	C57BL/6J	A/J	1–19, X, Y, M	Jackson Laboratory[a]
A/J-Chr Y$^{C57BL/6J}$	A/J	C57BL/6J	Y	Jackson Laboratory[a]
129-Chr19$^{MOLF/Ei}$	129S1/SvImJ	MOLF/Ei	19	J. Nadeau[b]
C57BL/6J-Chr1$^{129S1/SvImJ}$	C57BL/6J	129S1/SvImJ	7, 13, X, Y	J. Nadeau[b]
129S1/SvImJ$^{C57BL/6J}$	129S1/SvImJ	C57BL/6J	13, X, Y	J. Nadeau[b]
FVB/NJ-Chr7$^{I/LnJ}$	FVB/NJ	I/LnJ	7	K. Hunter[c]
FVB/NJ-Chr9$^{NZB/B1NJ}$		NZB/B1NJ	9	
FVB/NJ-Chr17$^{NZB/B1NJ}$		NZB/B1NJ	17	
FVB/NJ-Chr19$^{NZB/B1NJ}$		NZB/B1NJ	19	
C57BL/6J-Chr$^{MSM/Ms}$	C57BL/6J	MSM/Ms	Many	T. Shiroishi[d]
B6.Chr^{STF}	C57BL/6J	STF/Pas4	2, 6, 9, 10, 13, 14, 16, 19	X. Montagutelli[e]

[a]www.jax.org
[b]CSS@case.edu
[c]**ref. 47.**
[d]**ref. 41.**
[e]**ref. 40.**

Table 2
Available Congenic Strains Derived From Chromosome Substitution Strains (CSSs)

CSS Congenics	Host	Donor	Chromosome	Contact
C57BL/6J-Chr6[A/J]	C57BL/6	A/J	6	J. Nadeau[a]
C57BL/6J-Chr17[A/J]	C57BL/6	A/J	17	J. Nadeau[a]

[a]CSS@case.edu

7. Wang, X., Korstanje, R., Higgins, D., and Paigen, B. (2004) Haplotype analysis in multiple crosses to identify a QTL gene. *Genome Res.* **14,** 1767–1772.

8. Adams, D. J., Dermitzakis, E. T., Cox, T., et al. (2005) Complex haplotypes, copy number polymorphisms and coding variation in two recently divergent mouse strains. *Nat. Genet.* **37,** 532–536.

9. Shifman, S. and Darvasi, A. (2005) Mouse inbred strain sequence information and yin-yang crosses for quantitative trait locus fine mapping. *Genetics* **169,** 849–854.

10. Glazier, A. M., Nadeau, J. H., and Aitman, T. J. (2002) Finding genes that underlie complex traits. *Science* **298,** 2345–2349.

11. Brockmann, G. A. and Bevova, M. R. (2002) Using mouse models to dissect the genetics of obesity. *Trends Genet.* **18,** 367–376.

12. Abiola, O., Angel, J. M., Avner, P., et al. (2003) The nature and identification of quantitative trait loci: a community's view. *Nat. Rev. Genet.* **4,** 911–916.

13. Flint, J. (2003) Analysis of quantitative trait loci that influence animal behavior. *J. Neurobiol.* **54,** 46–77.

14. Flint, J., Valdar, W., Shifman, S., and Mott, R. (2005) Strategies for mapping and cloning quantitative trait genes in rodents. *Nat. Rev. Genet.* **6,** 271–286.

15. Snell, G. D. (1948) Methods for study of histocompatibility genes. *J. Genet.* **49,** 87–108.

16. Bailey, D. W. (1971) Recombinant-inbred strains. An aid to finding identity, linkage, and function of histocompatibility and other genes. *Transplantation* **11,** 325–327.

17. Taylor, B. A. (1978) Recombinant inbred strains: use in gene mapping, in *Origins of Inbred Mice,* (Morse, III, H.C., ed.), Academic Press, NY, pp. 423–438.

18. Darvasi, A., and Soller, M. (1995) Advanced intercross lines, an experimental population for fine genetic mapping. *Genetics* **141,** 1199–1207.

19. Valdar, W. S., Flint, J., and Mott, R. (2003) QTL fine-mapping with recombinant-inbred heterogeneous stocks and in vitro heterogeneous stocks. *Mamm. Genome* **14,** 830–838.

20. Nadeau, J. H., Singer, J. B., Matin, A., and Lander, E. S. (2000) Analysing complex genetic traits with chromosome substitution strains. *Nat. Genet.* **24,** 221–225.

21. Silver, L.M. (1995) *Mouse Genetics: Concepts and Applications,* Oxford University Press, Oxford.

22. Markel, P., Shu, P., Ebeling, C., et al. (1997) Theoretical and empirical issues for marker-assisted breeding of congenic mouse strains. *Nat. Genet.* **17,** 280–284.

23. Paigen, K. and Eppig, J. T. (2000) A mouse phenome project. *Mamm. Genome* **11,** 715–717.
24. Bogue, M. (2003) Mouse Phenome Project: understanding human biology through mouse genetics and genomics. *J. Appl. Physiol.* **95,** 1335–1337.
25. Bogue, M. A. and Grubb, S. C. (2004) The Mouse Phenome Project. *Genetica* **122,** 71–74.
26. Singer, J. B., Hill, A. E., Burrage, L. C., et al. (2004) Genetic dissection of complex traits with chromosome substitution strains of mice. *Science* **304,** 445–448.
27. Broman, K. W., Rowe, L. B., Churchill, G. A., and Paigen, K. (2002) Crossover interference in the mouse. *Genetics* **160,** 1123–1131.
28. Kruglyak, L. and Lander, E. S. (1995) A nonparametric approach for mapping quantitative trait loci. *Genetics* **139,** 1421–1428.
29. Doerge, R. W. and Churchill, G. A. (1996) Permutation tests for multiple loci affecting a quantitative character. *Genetics* **142,** 285–294.
30. Belknap, J. K. (2003) Chromosome substitution strains: some quantitative considerations for genome scans and fine mapping. *Mamm. Genome* **14,** 723–732.
31. Mather, K. (1949) *Biometrical Genetics,* Methuen, London.
32. Mather, K. and Harrison, B. J. (1949) The manifold effects of selection. *Heredity* **3,** 1–52.
33. Mather, K. and Harrison, B. J. (1949) The manifold effects of selection. *Heredity* **3,** 131–162.
34. Kuspira, J. and Unrau, J. (1957) Genetic analysis of certain characteristics in common wheat using whole chromosome substitution lines. *Can. J. Plant Sci.* **37,** 300–326.
35. Seiger, M. B. (1966) The effects of chromosome substitution on male body weight of Drosophila melanogaster. *Genetics* **53,** 237–248.
36. Matin, A., Collin, G. B., Asada, Y., Varnum, D., and Nadeau, J. H. (1999) Susceptibility to testicular germ-cell tumours in a 129.MOLF-Chr 19 chromosome substitution strain. *Nat. Genet.* **23,** 237–240.
37. Youngren, K. K., Nadeau, J. H., and Matin, A. (2003) Testicular cancer susceptibility in the 129.MOLF-Chr19 mouse strain: additive effects, gene interactions and epigenetic modifications. *Hum. Mol. Genet.* **12,** 389–398.
38. Collin, G. B., Asada, Y., Varnum, D. S., and Nadeau, J. H. (1996) DNA pooling as a quick method for finding candidate linkages in mutligenic trait analysis: an example involving susceptibility to germ cell tumors. *Mamm. Genome* **7,** 68–70.
39. Matin, A. and Nadeau, J. H. (2001) Sensitized polygenic trait analysis. *Trends Genet.* **17,** 727–731.
40. Santos, J., Montagutelli, X., Acevedo, A., et al. (2002) A new locus for resistance to gamma radiation-induced thymic lymphoma identified using inter-specific consomic and inter-specific recombinant congenic strains of mice. *Oncogene* **21,** 6680–6683.
41. Oka, A., Mita, A., Sakurai-Yamatani, N., et al. (2004) Hybrid breakdown caused by substitution of the X chromosome between two mouse subspecies. *Genetics* **166,** 913–924.

42. Petryshen, T. L., Kirby, A., Hammer, R. P., et al. (2005) Two QTLs for prepulse inhibition of startle identified on mouse chromosome 16 using chromosome substitution strains. *Genetics* **171,** 1895–1904.

43. Ackerman, K. G., Huang, H., Grasemann, H., et al. (2005) Interacting genetic loci cause airway hyperresponsiveness. *Physiol. Genomics* **21,** 105–111.

44. Poirier, C., Qin, Y., Adams, C. P., et al. (2004) A complex interaction of imprinted and maternal-effect genes modifies sex determination in Odd Sex (***Ods***) mice. *Genetics* **168,** 1557–1562.

45. Singer, J. B., Hill, A. E., Nadeau, J. H., and Lander, E. S. (2005) Mapping quantitative trait loci for anxiety in chromosome substitution strains of mice. *Genetics* **169,** 855–862.

46. Krewson, T. D., Supelak, P. J., Hill, A. E., et al. (2004) Chromosomes 6 and 13 harbor genes that regulate pubertal timing in mouse chromosome substitution strains. *Endocrinology* **145,** 4447–4451.

47. Lancaster, M., Rouse, J., and Hunter, K. W. (2005) Modifiers of mammary tumor progression and metastasis on mouse Chromosome 7, 9, and 17. *Mamm. Genome* **16,** 120–126.

48. Malek, R. L., Wang, H. Y., Kwitek, A. E., et al. (2006) Physiogenomic resources for rat models of heart, lung, and blood disorders. *Nat. Genet.* **38,** 234–239.

49. Cowley, A. W., Roman, R. J., and Jacob, H. J. (2003) Application of chromosomal substitution techniques in gene-function discovery. *J. Physiol.* **554,** 46–55.

50. Cowley, A. W., Liang, M., Roman, R. J., Greene, A. S., and Jacob, H. J. (2004) Consomic rat model systems for physiological genomics. *Acta Physiol. Scand.* **181,** 585–592.

12

Genome-Wide Association Study to Identify Single-Nucleotide Polymorphisms Conferring Risk of Myocardial Infarction

Kouichi Ozaki and Toshihiro Tanaka

Summary

Myocardial infarction (MI) is characterized by abrupt occlusion of coronary artery resulting in irreversible damage to cardiac muscle. This disease might result from the interactions of multiple genetic and environmental factors, none of which can cause disease solely by themselves. To reveal the genetic bases of MI, we performed a large-scale, case–control association study using 92,788 gene-based single-nucleotide polymorphism (SNP) markers. We have identified functional SNPs within the lymphotoxin-α gene located on chromosome 6p21 conferred susceptibility to MI. This chapter describes a detailed protocol for performing a genome-wide association study as used in our MI study.

Key Words: Myocardial infarction; single-nucleotide polymorphisms; SNPs; association study; high-throughput multiplex PCR-invader assay.

1. Introduction

Despite the changes in lifestyle and development of new pharmacological approaches, coronary artery disease including myocardial infarction (MI) continues to be the principal cause of death in many countries *(1,2)*, indicating the importance of identifying genetic and environmental factors in the pathogenesis of the disease. Common genetic variants are widely believed to contribute significantly to genetic risks of common diseases *(3–5)*. Although it is known that coronary risk factors, such as diabetes mellitus, hypercholesterolemia, and hypertension, have genetic components, a positive family history is an independent predictor, which suggests a genetic background of its own *(6)*. In recent years, candidate MI susceptibility genes were identified on several chromosome loci by using linkage analysis and/or single-nucleotide polymorphisms (SNPs) case–control association studies *(7–10)*.

From: *Methods in Molecular Medicine, Vol. 128: Cardiovascular Disease; Methods and Protocols; Volume 1*
Edited by: Q. Wang © Humana Press Inc., Totowa, NJ

Association-based methods using common variants as markers will be more powerful than linkage-based approaches for localization of genes related to such diseases, because linkage-based methods have low power to detect genes that exert only modest effects on a given process. For genome-wide association studies to succeed in identifying genes related to common diseases, linkage disequilibrium (LD)-based and haplotype-based mapping must define critical regions. Recent efforts of the haplotype analyses in the International HapMap Project *(11,12)*, which genotyped 600,000 SNPs, will provide more insight into marker–trait association studies.

To facilitate systematic analyses, we established a screening system to explore SNPs located within exons, introns, and promoter regions, because they might directly affect expression levels or protein functions of the corresponding genes. To date, this effort has identified approx 190,000 gene-based SNPs throughout the human genome (http://snp.ims.u-tokyo.ac.jp) *(13)*. In addition, we have developed a high-throughput SNP genotyping system using multiplex PCR invader technology (Third Wave Technologies, Madison, WI) that will enable us to type more than 100 million SNPs in 1 yr *(14)*. Using these resources and techniques, we have performed a genome-wide case–control association study to search for genes related to the pathogenesis of MI *(15)*.

2. Materials

2.1. Subjects (15)

The diagnosis of definite MI required two of the following three criteria: (1) a clinical history of central chest pressure, pain, or tightness lasting for 30 min or more, (2) ST-segment elevation greater than 0.1 mV in at least one standard or two precordial leads, and (3) a rise in the serum creatine kinase concentration to greater than twice the normal laboratory value. The control subjects consisted of the general population who were recruited through several medical institutes in Japan. All subjects were Japanese and gave written informed consent to participate in the study, according to the process approved by the Ethical Committee at SNP Research Center, The Institute of Physical and Chemical Research (RIKEN), Tokyo. Their parents gave their consent when the participants were under 16 yr old.

2.2. Preparation of Genomic DNA From Peripheral Blood Leukocyte

1. RBC lysis buffer: 10 mM NH$_4$HCO$_3$, 144 mM NH$_4$Cl (sterilize by autoclaving for 20 min at 15 psi [1.05 kb/cm^2] on liquid cycle).
2. Proteinase K buffer: 50 mM Tris-HCl, 100 mM NaCl, 1 mM EDTA (sterilize by autoclaving).
3. Proteinase K (Boehringer Mannheim) is dissolved at 10 mg/mL in TE buffer. Proteinase K must be self-digested by incubating at 37°C for 1 h.

4. 10% (w/v) sodium dodecyl sulfate (SDS) (filtrate by PALL 0.45 μm Acrodisc Syringefilter).
5. 8 *M* CH₃COONH₄ (sterilize by autoclaving).
6. TE buffer: 10 m*M* Tris-HCl, pH 8.0, 1 m*M* EDTA, pH 8.0 (1 *N* NaOH).

2.3. Multiplex PCR

1. Primers: we used the sequences for primers from our own SNP database, which is available on our website (http://snp.ims.u-tokyo.ac.jp).
2. Ex-Taq DNA polymerase (Takara Shuzo, Otsu, Japan).
3. 10X PCR buffer: 166 m*M* (NH₄)₂SO₄, 670 m*M* Tris-HCl, pH 8.8, 20 m*M* MgCl₂, 100 m*M* β-mercaptoethanol, 67 m*M* EDTA.
4. 78 m*M* MgCl₂.
5. Taq start antibody (Clontech Laboratories, Palo Alto, CA).
6. 25 m*M* dNTPs (TOYOBO, Osaka, Japan).
7. GeneAmp PCR system 9700 (Applied Biosystems, Foster City, CA).

2.4. Invader Assay

1. All reagents (reaction buffer, fluorescent resonance energy transfer [FRET] probe, allele-specific probe, enzyme, and so on) for the invader assay were supplied by Third Wave Technologies.
2. ABI7900 Sequence Detector (Applied Biosystems).

2.5. Statistical Analysis

Microsoft Excel software, SNP analyzer software (DYNACOM, Chiba, Japan).

3. Methods

As the first step of our comprehensive association study, we performed genotyping of 94 patients with MI by the high-throughput multiplex PCR invader assay method *(14)* using 92,788 gene-based SNPs *(13)* and compared the results with the allelic frequencies found in the 658 general Japanese individuals. The cutoff *p* value of 0.01 for association in either recessive or dominant models was used for this screening. We further genotyped SNPs that showed a *p* value of less than 0.01 in a larger replication panel of patients with MI and control subjects.

3.1. Extraction of Genomic DNA From Blood Cells (see Notes 1 and 2)

1. Collect 10 mL of fresh blood in tubes containing 1.75 mL of EDTA (*see* **Note 3**).
2. Transfer the collected blood to a 50-mL falcon tube (Beckton Dickinson Co.) and centrifuge at 1300*g* (3000 rpm in Beckman, CS-15R [rotor S4180]) for 5 min at room temperature. Remove the supernatant fluid by aspiration.
3. Add 30 mL RBC lysis buffer to the pellet fluid, vortex the tube, and incubate 20 min at room temperature.

4. Centrifuge at 1750*g* (3000 rpm in Beckman, CS-15R [rotor S4180]) for 5 min at room temperature. Remove the supernatant fluid by aspiration (*see* **Note 4**).
5. Repeat **steps 3** and **4** two times. White blood cells are obtained as a pellet.
6. Add 4 mL of proteinase K buffer to the pellet, vortex, and transfer the pellet to polypropylene tube.
7. Add 200 μL of 10% SDS and mix the solution gently five to six times.
8. Add 200 μL of proteinase K and mix the solution gently five to six times.
9. Store the solution at 37°C overnight.
10. Add 4 mL of phenol (equilibrated with 0.5 *M* Tris-HCl, pH 8.0).
11. Rotate the solution overnight (TAITEC; Rotator T-50; 1 turn/6–8 s).
12. By centrifugation at 1750*g* for 10 min at room temperature, the solution separates two phases (upper and lower phases) into equal volumes.
13. Using a wide-bore pipet, transfer the viscous aqueous phase to a fresh centrifuge tube.
14. Add an equal volume of phenol:chloroform:isoamyl alcohol (25:24:1).
15. Repeat **steps 11** and **12**.
16. Add an equal volume of chloroform:isoamyl alcohol (24:1).
17. Repeat **steps 11** and **12**.
18. Add 0.1 vol of 8 *M* CH$_3$COONH$_4$. Add an equal volume of isopropyl alcohol and gently mix the solution. The genomic DNA forms a precipitate.
19. Remove the precipitate in one piece from the solution with a Pasteur pipet whose end has been sealed and shaped into an "L."
20. Wash the DNA precipitate twice with 70% ethanol, and collect the DNA by centrifugation at 5000*g*.
21. Remove as much 70% ethanol as possible using an aspirator. Store the pellet of genomic DNA in an open tube at room temperature until the last visible trace of ethanol has evaporated. Do not allow the pellet of genomic DNA to dry completely, because desiccated DNA is very difficult to dissolve.
22. Add 0.5 mL of TE buffer (pH 8.0). Store the tube at 4°C overnight until the genomic DNA has completely dissolved. Store the genomic DNA solution at 4°C.

3.2. A Hundred Multiplex PCR

To reduce dimerization of primers and to increase the efficiency of PCR reaction, anti-taq antibody is used.

1. Combine the following volume of reagents:

    10X PCR buffer, 5 μL
    78 m*M* MgCl$_2$, 3 μL
    100 p*M* Each forward primer, 0.05 μL
    100 p*M* Each reverse primer, 0.05 μL
    Ex-Taq DNA polymerase (5 U/μL), 2 μL
    Taq start, 0.55 μg
    Genomic DNA, 40 ng
    Distilled water, up to 50 μL

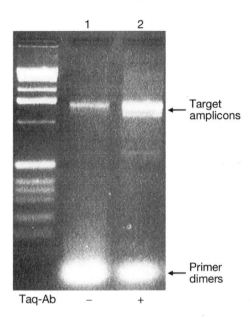

Fig. 1. A hundred multiplex PCR products without (lane 1) and with (lane 2) anti-Taq polymerase antibody (Taq-Ab). (Reproduced with permission from **ref. *14*.**)

2. Amplify the samples in Gene Amp PCR system 9700 using the following program:

     94°C for 2 min
     35 cycles
     94°C for 15 s
     60°C for 45 s
     72°C for 3 min

As shown **Fig. 1**, by addition of anti-Taq antibody, the PCR efficiency is significantly increased.

3.3. Genotyping by Invader Assay

The invader assay combines structure-specific cleavage enzymes and a universal FRET system.

1. Combine the following volume of reagents:

     Signal buffer, 0.5 µL
     FRET probe, 0.5 µL
     Structure-specific cleavage enzyme, 0.5 µL
     Allele-specific probe mix, 1 µL
     PCR products diluted 1:10, 2 µL
     Distilled water, 5.5 µL

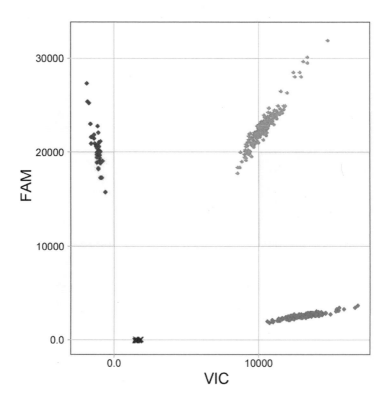

Fig. 2. Allelic discrimination of multiplex PCR products.

2. Incubate the samples at 95°C for 5 min, and then at 63°C 15 min (*see* **Note 5**).
3. Detect the signal using the ABI7900 Sequence Detector.

As shown in **Fig. 2**, alleles could be discriminated at a glance. **Fig. 3** shows the flow-chart of our high-throughput genotyping system.

3.4. Statistical Analyses for Genotyped SNPs

1. Assess Hardy-Weinberg Equilibrium (HWE) of alleles at individual loci by conventional χ^2 test, and exclude the SNPs that are deviated from HWE (we generally use a cutoff p value of 0.01 for deviation of HWE).
2. Using conventional χ^2 test, calculate the p value for association in either dominant or recessive models for the screening.
3. Choose the SNPs that had p values of less than 0.01, and genotype in a larger replication panel of individuals with MI and control subjects (we generally genotype a total of 1000 MI samples and 1000 control samples).
4. Choose the SNPs that had p values of less than 10^{-6}, and further analyze the dense SNPs map of the SNPs loci for haplotype structure, followed by functional analyses of the gene products with SNPs.

Procedure	Genomic DNA
Multiplex PCR	

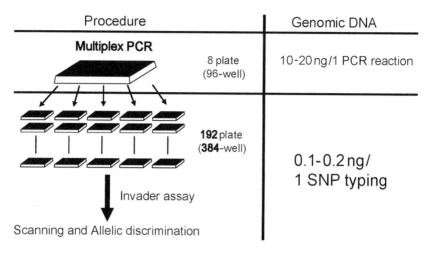

Fig. 3. Experimental flow-chart-chart for invader assay procedure, after the simultaneous PCR amplification of 100 genomic fragments, also showing the calculated amount of DNA required in each step. (Reproduced with permission from **ref. *14*.**)

4. Notes

1. To obtain a pure high-molecular-weight genomic DNA, avoid a mechanical breakage of DNA due to strong vortexing of the DNA solution.
2. To avoid a contamination of cloned DNA (i.e., plasmid DNA), use an exclusive room for genomic DNA.
3. Do not use heparin as an anticoagulant; heparin prevents a PCR reaction.
4. For decontamination, the liquid waste must be treated with appropriate reagent (i.e., HOCl) or autoclave.
5. The reaction time (63°C) is dependent on fluorescent signal density. If one can not obtain a discrimination of alleles (major homozygote, heterozygote, and minor homozygote), reaction time should be expanded (~90 min).

References

1. Breslow, J. L. (1997) Cardiovascular disease burden increases, NIH funding decreases. *Nature Med.* **3,** 600–601.
2. Braunwald, E. (1997) Shattuck lecture—cardiovascular medicine at the turn of the millennium: triumphs, concerns, and opportunities. *N. Engl. J. Med.* **337,** 1360–1369.
3. Risch, N. and Merikangas, K. (1996) The future of genetic studies of complex human diseases. *Science* **273,** 1516–1517.
4. Collins, F. S., Guyer, M. S., and Charkravarti, A. (1997) Variations on a theme: cataloging human DNA sequence variation. *Science* **278,** 1580–1581.
5. Lander, E. S. (1996) The new genomics: global views of biology. *Science* **274,** 536–539.

6. Marenberg, M. E., Risch, N., Berkman, L. F., Floderus, B., and de Faire, U. (1994) Genetic susceptibility to death from coronary heart disease in a study of twins. *N. Engl. J. Med.* **330,** 1041–1046.

7. Yamada, Y., Izawa, H., Ichihara, S., et al. (2002) Prediction of the risk of myocardial infarction from polymorphisms in candidate genes. *N. Engl. J. Med.* **347,** 1916–1923.

8. Wang, L., Fan, C., Topol, S. E., Topol, E. J., and Wang, Q. (2003) Mutation of MEF2A in an inherited disorder with features of coronary artery disease. *Science* **302,** 1578–1581.

9. Helgadottir, A., Manolescu, A., Thorleifsson, G., et al. (2004) The gene encoding 5-lipoxygenase activating protein confers risk of myocardial infarction and stroke. *Nat. Genet.* **36,** 233–239.

10. Cipollone, F., Toniato, E., Martinotti, S., et al. (2004) A polymorphism in the cyclooxygenase 2 gene as an inherited protective factor against myocardial infarction and stroke. *JAMA* **291,** 2221–2228.

11. The international HapMap consortium. (2003) The International HapMap Project. *Nature* **426,** 789–796.

12. The International HapMap Consortium. (2004) Integrating ethics and science in the international HAPMAP project. *Nat. Rev. Genet.* **5,** 467–475.

13. Haga, H., Yamada, R., Ohnishi, Y., Nakamura, Y., and Tanaka, T. (2002) Gene-based SNP discovey as part of the Japanese Millennium Genome project: identification of 190,562 genetic variations in the human genome. *J. Hum. Genet.* **47,** 605–610.

14. Ohnishi, Y., Tanaka, T. Ozaki, K., Yamada, R., Suzuki, H., and Nakamura, Y. (2001) A high-throughput SNP typing system for genome-wide association studies. *J. Hum. Genet.* **46,** 471–477.

15. Ozaki, K., Ohnishi, Y., Iida, A., et al. (2002) Functional SNPs in the lymphotoxin-alpha gene that are associated with susceptibility to myocardial infarction. *Nature Genet.* **32,** 650–654.

13

Mutation Detection in Congenital Long QT Syndrome

Cardiac Channel Gene Screen Using PCR, dHPLC, and Direct DNA Sequencing

David J. Tester, Melissa L. Will, and Michael J. Ackerman

Summary

Within the field of molecular cardiac electrophysiology, the previous decade of research elucidated the fundamental genetic substrate underlying many arrhythmogenic disorders such as long QT syndrome (LQTS), catecholaminergic polymorphic ventricular tachycardia (CPVT), Andersen-Tawil syndrome, Brugada Syndrome, and Timothy syndrome. In addition, the genetic basis for cardiomyopathic processes vulnerable to sudden arrhythmic death—hypertrophic cardiomyopathy, dilated cardiomyopathy, and arrhythmogenic right ventricular cardiomyopathy—are understood now in greater detail.

The majority of congenital LQTS is understood as a primary cardiac channelopathy that often but not always provides evidence of its presence via a prolonged QT interval on the 12-lead surface electrocardiogram. To date, more than 300 mutations have been identified in five genes encoding key ion channel subunits involved in the orchestration of the heart's action potential. LQTS genetic testing has been performed in research laboratories over the past decade, relying on the techniques of PCR, an intermediate mutation analysis platform such as single-stranded conformation polymorphism (SSCP) or denaturing high-performance liquid chromatography (dHPLC), and subsequent direct DNA sequencing to elucidate the genetic underpinnings of this disorder. Presently, LQTS genetic testing is a clinically available molecular diagnostic test that provides comprehensive open reading frame/splice site mutational analysis via high-throughput DNA sequencing. This chapter will focus on LQTS genetic testing employing the techniques of genomic DNA isolation from peripheral blood, exon-specific PCR amplification, dHPLC heteroduplex analysis, and direct DNA sequencing.

Key Words: Long QT syndrome; cardiac ion channels; genetic testing; DNA isolation; PCR; denaturing high-performance liquid chromatography; dHPLC; DNA sequencing; mutations.

From: *Methods in Molecular Medicine, Vol. 128: Cardiovascular Disease; Methods and Protocols; Volume 1*
Edited by: Q. Wang © Humana Press Inc., Totowa, NJ

1. Introduction

Congenital long QT syndrome (LQTS) is a potentially lethal arrhythmogenic disorder characterized by abnormal repolarization of the myocardium that may manifest on the surface electrocardiogram as a prolonged QT interval. LQTS causes syncope, seizures, or sudden death, as a result of recurrent or lethal arrhythmias (torsades de pointes) usually following a precipitating event such as exertion, emotion, or auditory stimuli.

At a molecular level, LQTS is generally understood as a cardiac channelopathy with a plethora of mutations identified in five genes encoding critical ion channel proteins subunits: *KCNQ1/KVLQT1*, *KCNH2/HERG*, *SCN5A*, *KCNE1/MinK*, and *KCNE2/MiRP1* (*1–6*). Together, these genes are comprised of 60 amino acid translating exons and constitute the LQTS cardiac channel gene screen that has been performed by research laboratories over the past decade and the present-day clinical diagnostic test. To date, hundreds of unique mutations in these LQTS-causing genes have been discovered in 75% of clinically robust LQTS families investigated. Missense mutations are the most common (72%) type of mutation found, whereas frameshift (insertion and deletion) mutations (10%), in-frame deletions, and nonsense and splice-site mutations (5–7% each) account for the remaining types of mutations in LQTS (*3,4*). The mutations are scattered throughout the coding sequences of the five genes and there do not appear to be any particular "hot-spots" where mutations are concentrated. Approximately 5–10% of cases host multiple LQTS-associated mutations, with some of these multiples occurring in more than one gene (i.e., the presence of a *KCNQ1* plus a *KCNH2* mutation in the same individual) (*4*). As a result of the heterogeneous nature of LQTS, a comprehensive mutational analysis of all five-channel genes is highly recommended when performing genetic testing for this disorder. This chapter will focus on the analysis of the cardiac channel genes implicated in the more standard Romano-Ward (autosomal-dominant) version of LQTS. Analysis for mutations in the *ANKB*-encoded ankyrin B (LQT4), *KCNJ2*-encoded Kir2.1 potassium channel (ATS1), and the *CACNA1C*-encoded L-type calcium channel alpha subunit (TS1) are beyond the scope of this chapter.

The identification of gene mutations typically involves the PCR technique used to amplify many copies of a specific region of DNA sequence within the gene of interest. Generally, 20- to 25-bp forward and reverse oligonucleotide primers are designed within intronic DNA sequences flanking the exon (amino acid encoding) of interest in order to produce PCR products (200–400 bp in length) containing the desired exon to be analyzed. In cases of large exons, overlapping PCR products may need to be designed. Briefly, a genomic DNA sample isolated from blood or tissue is combined with both a forward and reverse amplification primer specific for the region of desired amplification (usually an entire exon) along with a reaction mixture containing dinucleotides (dATP, dCTP, dGTP, and dTTP) or "DNA building blocks" and a DNA polymerase. The reaction mixture is subjected to cycling (typically 30–40 cycles) of specific temperatures designed to: denature (95°C) double stranded DNA, allow for primer annealing (typically at 55–62°C), and to elongate (72°C) the newly synthesized DNA strand. A well-optimized PCR reaction will yield millions of copies of the specific sequence of interest. These PCR products can be used in many downstream molecular techniques.

PCR amplification is often followed by the use of an intermediate mutation detection platform such as denaturing high performance liquid chromatography (dHPLC). dHPLC is one of the most sensitive and accurate technologies for the elucidation of unknown gene mutations *(7,8)*. The technique is used to inform the investigator of the presence or absence of a DNA sequence change in the samples examined. dHPLC is based on the formation and separation of double-stranded DNA fragments containing a mismatch in the base pairing between the "wild-type" and "mutant" DNA strands, known as heteroduplex DNA. In general, PCR products are subjected to denaturing (heating) and reannealing (cooling) in order to form heteroduplex (mismatch) and homoduplex (perfect match) molecular species **(Fig. 1A)**. If a sample contains a heterozygous mutation, then heteroduplex and homoduplex fragments will be produced following this denaturing and re-annealing procedure. If a sample is "wild-type" or homozygous, then only homoduplex fragments will be produced **(Fig. 1A)**. The crude PCR products are injected on to a solid phase column that is heated to a specific temperature (individually optimized for each unique PCR product) that allows for partial denaturing of the DNA sequence of interest. A linear acetonitrile gradient based on the size of the PCR product is applied to the column to flush the DNA strands and send the PCR products through an ultraviolet (UV) detector resulting in a chromatogram showing the sample's elution profile. This elution profile is highly reproducible under optimal conditions. Because heteroduplex species are less thermodynamically stable than homoduplexes, these double-stranded complexes will begin to unravel at the elevated temperature and elute from the column sooner then their homoduplex or "wild-type" counter parts, thus producing an elution profile that is different from the "wild-type" profile, and allowing for detection of mutation harboring samples. Specifically, PCR products containing heterozygote mutations result in the presence of profiles with "shouldering" or additional "peaks" as when compared with "wild-type" samples **(Fig. 1B)**.

Although intermediate mutation detection platforms inform the investigator of which samples contain mutations, direct DNA sequencing must be used to decipher the precise underlying DNA change(s). Many large biomedical insti-

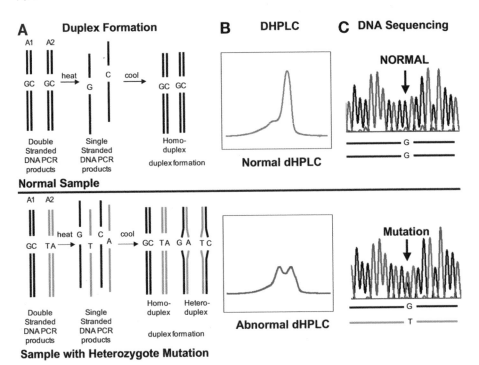

Fig. 1. Mutation detection process of PCR, denaturing high-performance liquid chromatography (dHPLC), and DNA sequencing. Mutation detection by dHPLC relies on heteroduplex (mismatch) and homoduplex (perfect match) formation by heating and cooling of both DNA alleles (**A1,A2**) and then separating such species by ion-exchange chromatography resulting in (**B**) dHPLC elution profiles that differ from normal profiles. (**C**) DNA sequencing is then used to determine the underlying heterozygote DNA change.

tutions have DNA sequencing core facilities where the investigator can submit a normal control sample along with samples of interest for analysis. The method illustrated in this chapter was kindly provided by our sequencing core facility. Typically, PCR products to be sequenced are purified from the unincorporated amplification primers and dinucleotides (dNTP) using either an enzymatic or filter column-based technique. Pure PCR products are then subjected to sequencing using a single-oligonucleotide primer (usually the same forward amplification primer used in the original PCR reaction) and a sequencing reaction mixture containing a sequencing DNA polymerase, dinucleotides (dNTP), and dye-labeled dideoxynucleotides (ddATP-green, ddCTP-blue, ddGTP-black, and ddTTP-red). This mixture of sequencing reaction components and PCR product templates are cycled through a series of temperatures similar to that seen in a typical PCR reaction. Resulting sequencing products are then separated according to size by gel-based or capillary-based electrophoresis and a sequencing chromatogram is produced (**Fig. 1C**).

Review and comparison of the resulting sequence chromatograms and the published "wild-type" DNA and amino acid sequence for the gene/protein of interest will allow for the interpretation of whether the underlying DNA change is protein-altering and potentially pathogenic or a nonpathogenic normal variant. It is imperative that extreme caution be exercised with respect to the assignment of a variant as a pathogenic LQTS-causing mutation. Ethnically matched controls must be employed. We have recently provided the first comprehensive determination of the spectrum and prevalence of nonsynonymous single-nucleotide polymorphisms (SNPs) (i.e., amino acid substitutions) in the five LQTS-associated cardiac ion channel genes in approx 800 healthy control subjects from four distinct ethnic groups *(9,10)*. Approximately 2–5% of healthy individuals were found to host a rare variant. This compendium may serve as a molecular hit list of channel variants present within the normal population.

In this three-step approach—(1) PCR amplification, (2) dHPLC heterozygote analysis, and (3) DNA sequencing—only samples believed to contain a DNA change are further analyzed by DNA sequencing. In some cases, the use of an intermediate mutation detection platform such as dHPLC is bypassed for direct DNA sequencing of all samples interrogated. Although this approach to mutational analysis is very expensive, it may accelerate mutation detection.

2. Materials

2.1. DNA Isolation

1. Purgene Blood DNA isolation kit from Gentra Systems (Minneapolis, MN).
2. 100% Isopropanol.
3. 70% Ethanol.

2.2. PCR (see Table 1)

1. GenAmp 10 PCR buffer II (Applied Biosystems, Foster City, CA): 100 mM Tris-HCl, pH 8.3, 500 mM KCl.
2. 100 mM (pH 7.0) solutions of dATP, dCTP, dGTP, and dTTP.
3. Sterile H_2O, 18 Ω-cm.
4. Prepare 1 mL of 5X PCR buffer by adding 25 μL of each dNTP to 500 μL of 10X PCR buffer and 400 μL of sterile 18 Ω-cm H_2O. Mix by vortexing (*see* **Note 1**).
5. 25 mM MgCl$_2$ (Applied Biosystems).
6. Dimethylsulfoxide (DMSO), ACS grade.
7. Glycerol.
8. Prepare a 50% solution of glycerol: pour 25 mL of glycerol into a 50-mL polypropylene tube and fill with sterile 18 Ω-cm H_2O. Mix by vortexing.

Table 1
Recipe for PCR

Reaction mixture	1	Master mix		
		1	5	106
Sterile 18 Ω-cm H_2O	10.6	53	1123.6	
5X PCR buffer	4	20	424	
$MgCl_2$ (25 mM)	1.6	8	169.6	
Primer F (20 pmoles/µL)	0.8	4	84.8	
Primer R (20 pmoles/µL)	0.8	4	84.8	
Glycerol (50%)				
Formamide				
DMSO				
DNA (25 ng/µL)	2			
Ampli*taq* Gold (5 U/µL)	0.2	1	21.2	
Total volume	20			

9. Formamide.
10. Ampli*taq* Gold (5 U/µL) (Applied Biosystems).
11. HotStart Taq DNA Polymerase (5U/µL) (Qiagen, Valencia, CA) (*see* **Note 2**).
12. HotStart Taq 10X PCR buffer (containing 15 mM $MgCl_2$) (Qiagen) (*see* **Note 2**).
13. Oligonucleotide forward and reverse PCR primers (20 pmoles/µL) (**Tables 2–6**).
14. 0.2-mL Sterile individual or strip PCR reaction tubes with caps or 0.2-mL volume, 96-well thin-walled microplates with plate sealer for PCR applications.

2.3. Agarose Check Gel

1. 10X TBE: 0.89 M Tris borate, pH 8.3, 20 mM Na_2 EDTA.
2. Agarose 3:1 (Ameresco, Solon, OH).
3. Ethidium bromide (0.625 mg/mL).
4. 6X sample buffer: 0.25% Orange G, 15% Ficoll Type 400.
5. 18 Ω-cm H_2O.

2.4. Denaturing High-Performance Liquid Chromatography

1. HPLC-grade 2 M triethylammonium acetate (TEAA), pH 7.4 (Transgenomic, Omaha, NE).
2. HPLC-grade acetonitrile (ACN).
3. Prepare 1 L of buffer A (50 mM TEAA): using volumetric flasks, combine 50 mL of 2 M TEAA with 950 mL of 18 Ω-cm pure H_2O. Mix by inverting several times (*see* **Note 3**).
4. Prepare 1 L of buffer B (25% ACN, 50 mM TEAA): using volumetric flasks, combine 50 mL of 2 M TEAA and 250 mL of ACN with 700 mL of 18 Ω-cm pure H_2O. Mix by inverting several times (*see* **Note 3**).

Table 2
Oligonucleotide Primers and PCR and Denaturing High-Performance Liquid Chromatography (dHPLC) Conditions for Mutational Analysis of KCNQ1

Exon	Forward primer (5'–3')	Reverse primer (5'–3')	Size (bp)	$[MgCl_2]$ (mM)	Thermal cycling method	Gradient 1 (%B; temp °C)	Gradient 2 (%B; temp °C)
1a	CTCGCCTTCGCTGCAGCTC	GCGCGGGTCTAGGCTCACC	332	2[a]	2	58–68%; 70	52–62%; 73
1b	CGCCGCGCCCCAGTTGC	CAGAGCTCCCCACCACCAG	201	2[a]	2	55–65%; 66	51–61%; 70
2	ATGGGCAGAGGCGCGTGATGCTGAC	ATCCAGCCATGCCCTCAGATGC	165	1.5	1	51–61%; 64	
3	GTTCAAACAGGTTGCAGGGTCTGA	CTTCCTGGTCTGGAAACCTGG	222	2	1	54–64%; 65	50–60%; 68
4	CTCTTCCCTGGGGCCCTGGC	TGCGGGGGAGCTTGTGGCACAG	169	2	1	51–61%; 65	
5	TCAGCCCACACCATCTCCTTC	CTGGGCCCCTACCCTAACCC	151	2	1	50–60%; 64	
6	TCCTGGAGCCCGACACTGTGTGT	TGTCCTGCCCACTCCTCAGCCT	237	1.5	1	55–65%; 63	51–61%; 66
7	TGGCTGACCACTGTCCCTCT	CCCCAGGACCCCAGCTGTCCAA	195	1.5	1	53–63%; 64	
8	GCTGGCAGTGGCCTGTGTGGA	AACAGTGACCAAAATGACAGTGAC	191	2	1	49–59%; 66	
9	TGGCTCAGCAGGTGACAGC	TGGTGGCAGGTGGGCTACT	186	2	1	54–64%; 64	
10	GCCTGGCAGACGATGTCCA	CAACTGCCTGAGGGGTTCT	212	2	1	54–64%; 59	48–58%; 64
11	CTGTCCCCACACTTTCTCCT	TGAGCTCCAGTCCCCTCCAG	184	2	1	52–62%; 63	
12	TGGCCACTCACAATCTCCT	GCCTTGACACCCTCCACTA	155	2	1	52–62%; 64	
13	GGCACAGGGAGGAGAAGTG	CGGCACCGCTGATCATGCA	201	2	1	50–60%; 66.5	
14	CCAGGGCCAGGTGTGACTG	TGGGCCCAGAGTAACTGACA	120	2[b]	3	49–59%; 60	
15	CCTGATTTGGGTGTTTTATCC[c]	CACAGGGAGGTGCCTGCT[c]	135	2	1	49–59%; 60	47–57%; 65
16	CACCACTGACTCTCTCGTCT	CCATCCCCAGCCCCATC	298	1.5	1	57–67%; 66	53–63%; 68

dHPLC was performed using a 5% buffer B/minute gradient. The start and stop %B (buffer B) followed by the temperature at which the gradient was performed is indicated in the table.

[a] A final concentration of 10% glycerol and 4% formamide was added to the reaction mixture.
[b] A final concentration of 8% DMSO was added to the reaction mixture.
[c] Indicates primer sequences from the present study; all others are according to Splawski et al. (11).

Table 3
Oligonucleotide Primers and PCR and Denaturing High-Performance
Liquid Chromatography (dHPLC) Conditions for Mutational Analysis of KCNH2

Exon	Forward primer (5'-3')	Reverse primer (5'-3')	Size (bp)	[MgCl$_2$] (mM)	Thermal cycling method	Gradient 1 (%B; temp °C)	Gradient 2 (%B; temp °C)
1	CCGCCCATGGGCTCAGG	ATCCACACTCGGAAGAAGTC[a]	143	2[c]	2	51–61%; 66	44–54%; 70
2	CCCGCTCACGCGCACTCT[b]	ACCCCGCCCCGTGGTCGT[b]	308	1.5[d]	2	57–67%; 66	55–65%; 69
3	GGGCTATGTCCTCCCACTCT	AGCCTGCCTAAAGCAAGTACA	216	2	1	54–64%; 63	50–60%; 65
4a	ACGACCACGTGCCTCTCCTCT[a]	GGGACCCACCAGCGCACGCCG[a]	261	2[e]	2	56–66%; 69	51–61%; 72
4b	GCCATGGACAACCACGTGGCA	CCCAGAATGCAGCAAGCCTG	302	2[e]	2	55–65%; 71	
5	GGCCTGACCACGCTGCCTCT	CCCTCTCCAAGCTCCTCCA	287	2	1	57–67%; 63	53–63%; 65
6a	CAGAGATGTTCATCGCTCCTG	CAGGCGTAGCCACACTCGGTAG	292	2	1	57–67%; 65	51–61%; 67
6b	TTCCTGCTGAAGGAGGACGGAAG	TACACCACCTGCCTCCTTGCTGA	296	2	1	57–67%; 64	
7a	TGCCCATCAACGGAATGTGC	GAAGTAGAGCGCCGTCACATAC	333	2	1	56–66%; 66	54–64%; 68
7b	CAGCCACACATGGACTCAC[b]	AGTTTCCTCCAACTTGGGTTC	241	2	2	57–67%; 64	
8	GCAGAGGCTGACGGCCCCA	CAGCCTGCCACCCACTGG[b]	279	2	1	57–67%; 66	
9	ATGGTGGAGTGGAGTGTGGGTT	AGAAGGCTCGCACCTCTTGAG	331	2	2	58–68%; 65	
10	GAGAGGTGCCTGCTGCCTGG	ACAGCTGGAAGCAGGAGGATG	286	2	1	57–67%; 63	
11	ACCCCGGTGGGGCAGGAGAGCACTG[b]	CCTTCCAGCTCCCAGCCTCACCTTG[b]	241	1.5	2	52–62%; 63	48–58%; 65
12a	TGAGGCCCATTCTCTGTTTCC	CTTCTCGCAGTCTCCATCA[b]	271	1	2	53–63%;67	
12b	TGAGAGCAGTGAGGATGA[a]	TAGACGCACCACCGCTGCC[a]	210	1	2	54–64%;67	
13	CTCACCCAGCTCTGCTCTG	CACCAGGACCTGGACCAGACT	269	1	2	54–64%; 65	52–62%; 67
14	GTGGAGGCTGTCACTGGTGT	GAGGAAGCAGGGCTGGAGCTT	258	2	1	54–64%; 65	52–62%; 67
15	TGCCCATGCTCTGTGTGTATTG	CGGCCCAGCAGCGCCTTGATC	199	2	1	55–65%; 63	51–61%; 67

Primer sequences are according to Splawski et al. (11) except where otherwise noted: [a]ref. 14 and [b]primer sequences are according to the present study. dHPLC was performed using a 5% buffer B/minute gradient. The start and stop %B (buffer B) followed by the temperature at which the gradient was performed is indicated in the table.

[c]A final concentration of 8% DMSO was added to the reaction mixture.
[d]HotStart Taq polymerase was used rather than Amplitaq Gold.
[e]A final concentration of 10% glycerol and 4% formamide was added to the reaction mixture.
[d]Primer sequences are according to the present study.

Table 4

Oligonucleotide Primers and PCR and Denaturing High-Performance Liquid Chromatography (dHPLC) Conditions for Mutational Analysis of SCN5A

Exon	Forward primer (5'–3')	Reverse primer (5'–3')	Size (bp)	[MgCl$_2$] (mM)	Thermal cycling method	Gradient 1 (%B; temp °C)	Gradient 2 (%B; temp °C)
2	GGTCTGCCCACCTGCTCTCT	CCTCTTCCCCTCTGCTCCATT	326	2	1	52–62%; 66	52–62%; 68
3	AGTCCAAGGGCTCTGAGCCAA	GGTACTCAGCAGGTATTAACTGCAA	230	1^b	4	53–63%; 61	49–59%; 63
4	GGTAGCACTGTCCTGGCAGTGAT	CCTGGACTCAAGTCCCCTTC	290	2	1	57–67%; 63	
5	TCACTCCACGTAAGGAACCTG	ATGTGGACTGCAGGGAGGAAGC	172	2	1	56–66%; 63	
6	AAGATGCCCAGGTTTGCCTC^a	TTCTGGTGACAGGCACATTC^a	350	1.5	2	54–64%; 61	
7	CCACCTCTGGTTGCCTACACTG	GTCTGCGGTCTCACAAAGTCTTC	276	2	1	57–67%; 64	55–65%; 66
8	CGAGTGCCCCTCACCAGCATG	GGAGACTCCCCTGGCAGGACAA	150	2	1	50–60%; 61	
9	GGGAGACAAGTCCAGCCCAGCAA	AGCCCACACTTGCTGTCCCTTG	209	1^b	4	56–66%; 56	56–66%; 61
10	ACTTGGAAATGCCCTCACCCAGA	CACCTATAGGCACCATCAGTCAG	310	1.5^c	2	56–66%; 63	
11	AAACGTCCGTTCCTCCACTCT	AACCCACAGCTGGGATTACCATT	211	2	1	54–64%; 62	
12a	GCCAGTGGCTCAAAAGACACAGGCT	CCTGGGCACTGGTCCGGCGCA	258	2	1	54–64%; 64	50–60%; 66
12b	CACCACACTCACTGCTGGTGC	GGAACTGCTGATCAGTTTGGGAGA	280	2	1	55–65%; 65	53–63%; 66
13	CCCTTTTCCCCAGCTGACGCAAA	GTCTAAAGCAGGCCAAGACAAATG	300	2	1	51–61%; 66	
14	CAGGAAGGTATTCCAGTTACATATGA	ACCCATGAAGCTGTGCCAGCTGT	338	1^b	4	58–68%; 63	
15	CTTTCCTATCCCAAACAATACCT	CCCCACCATCCCCCATGCAGT	230	2	1	55–65%; 61	51–63%; 64
16	GAGCCAGAGACCTTCACAAGGTCCCCT	CCCTTGCCACTTACCACACAAG	351	2	1	57–67%; 63	
17a	GGGACTGGATGGCTTGGCATGGT	CGGGGAGTAGGGGTGGCAATG	250	1^b	4	56–66%; 64	51–61%; 67
17b	GCCCAGGGCCAGCTGCCCAGCT	CTGTATATGTAGGTGCCTTATACATG	285	1^b	4	53–63%; 65	
18	AGGGTCTAAACCCCCAGGGTCA	CCCAGCTGGCTTCAGGGACAAA	162	2	1	53–63%; 66	
19	GAGGCCAAAGGCTGCTACTCAG	CCTGTCCCCTCTGGGTGGAACT	209	2	1	58–68%; 64	
20	CTTCAACCATCCAACCTTCTGC	CAGTTTCTGACCTGACTTTCCA	335	2.0	2	57–67%; 59	56–66%; 64
21	TGGTCCAGGCTTCATGTC^a	TCCGCCTCAGCTCCTTCT^a	290	1.5^c	2	56–66%; 62	
22	AGTGGGGAGCTGTTCCCATCCT	GGACCGCCTCCCACTCC	162	2	1	53–63%; 64	49–59%; 66
23	TTGAAAAGGAAATGTGCTCTGGG	AACATCATGGGTGATGGCCAT	283	1.5^c	2	60–70%; 62	
24	CTCAAGCGAGGTACAGAATTAAATGA	GGGCTTTCAGATGCAGCACTGAT	104	1^b	4	51–61%; 59	47–57%; 63

(*continued*)

Table 4 (*Continued*)
Oligonucleotide Primers and PCR and Denaturing High-Performance
Liquid Chromatography (dHPLC) Conditions for Mutational Analysis of SCN5A

Exon	Forward primer (5'–3')	Reverse primer (5'–3')[a]	Size (bp)	[MgCl$_2$] (mM)	Thermal cycling method	Gradient 1 (%B; temp °C)	Gradient 2 (%B; temp °C)
25	GAGACCCCAGCCTGTCTGA[a]	TGGGACCTGCAGCCTGAGT[a]	253	2	1	56–66%; 59	50–60%; 62
26	GCTGGGGCCTCTGAGAAC	CACAAAACCAGGAGCCTGG	149	2	1	52–62%; 63	46–56%; 65
27	CCCAGCGAGCACTTTCCATTTG	GCTTCTCCGTCCAGCTGACTTGTA	316	2	1	60–70%; 60	
28a	TGCACAGTGATGCTGGCTGGAA	GAAGAGGCACAGCATGCTGTTGG	303	2	1	57–67%; 63	54–64%; 65
28b	AAGTGGGAGGCTGGCATCGAC	GTGCTCCTCCCGTGGCCACGC	301	2	1	57–67%; 62	51–61%; 66
28c	GAGCCCAGCCGTGGGCATCCT	GTCCCCACTCACCATGGGCAG	311	2	1	58–68%; 61	
28d	CCAACCAGATAAGCCTCATCAACA	CCGCCTGCTGACGGAAGAGGA	309	1[b]	4	53–63%; 64	
28e	TGCTCGAACGCTCTTTGAAGCAT	AAAGGCTGCTTTTCAGTGTGTCCT	345	2	1	58–68%; 63	53–63%; 65

Primer sequences are according to Wang et al. (*12*) except where otherwise noted: [a] primer sequences are according to the present study. dHPLC was performed using a 5% buffer B/minute gradient. The start and stop %B (buffer B) followed by the temperature at which the gradient was performed is indicated in the table.
[b] A final concentration of 8% DMSO was added to the reaction mixture.
[c] HotStarTaq polymerase was used rather than Amplitaq Gold.

Table 5
Oligonucleotide Primers and PCR and Denaturing High-Performance
Liquid Chromatography (dHPLC) Conditions for Mutational Analysis of KCNE1

Exon	Forward primer (5′–3′)	Reverse primer (5′–3′)	Size (bp)	[MgCl₂] (mM)	Thermal cycling method	Gradient 1 (%B; temp °C)	Gradient 2 (%B; temp °C)
3a	CTGCAGCAGTGGAACCTTAATG	GTTCGAGTGCTCCAGCTTCTTG	243	2	1	55–65%; 63	53–63%; 65
3b	GGGCATCATGCTGAGCTACAT	TTTAGCCAGTGGTGGGGTTCA	218	2	1	54–64%; 62	52–62%; 64

Primer sequences are according to Splawski et al. *(11)*. dHPLC was performed using a 5% buffer B/minute gradient. The start and stop %B (buffer B) followed by the temperature at which the gradient was performed is indicated in the table.

Table 6
Oligonucleotide Primers and PCR and Denaturing High-Performance
Liquid Chromatography (dHPLC) Conditions for Mutational Analysis of KCNE2

Exon	Forward primer (5'–3')	Reverse primer (5'—3')	Size (bp)	[MgCl$_2$] (mM)	Thermal cycling method	Gradient 1 (%B; temp °C)	Gradient 2 (%B; temp °C)
1a	CCGTTTTCCTAACCTTGTTCG	AGCATCAACTTTGGCTTGGAG	186	2 mM	2	52–62%; 58	48–58%; 60
1b	GTCTTCCGAAGGATTTTTATTAC	GTTCCCGTCTCTTGGATTTCA	196	2 mM	2	53–63%; 57	53–63%; 59
1c	AATGTTCTCTTTCATCATCGTG	TGTCTGGACGTCAGATGTTAG	239	2 mM	2	53–63%; 60	

Primer sequences are according to Abbott et al. (*13*). dHPLC was performed using a 5% buffer B/minute gradient. The start and stop %B (buffer B) followed by the temperature at which the gradient was performed is indicated in the table.

5. Prepare 1 L of syringe wash (buffer C) (8% ACN): dilute, in a volumetric flask, 80 mL of ACN with 18 Ω-cm H_2O. Mix by inverting several times (*see* **Note 3**).
6. Prepare 1 L of active wash (buffer D) (75% ACN): using a volumetric flask, combine 250 mL of 18 Ω-cm H_2O with 750 mL of ACN. Mix by inverting several times (*see* **Note 3**).
7. WAVE low-range mutation control standard (Transgenomic).
8. DNAsep HT Cartridge (Transgenomic).
9. In-line filters (Transgenomic).

2.5. PCR Product Purification

1. ExoSAP-it (exonuclease I, 10 U/mL and shrimp alkaline phosphatase, 2 U/mL) (USB, Cleveland, OH).

2.6. DNA Sequencing—Performed by Our Sequencing Core Facility

1. 18 Ω-cm H_2O.
2. Sequencing primer (2 pmol/μL): this is a 1/10 dilution of either the forward or reverse PCR amplification primer.
3. Big Dye Terminator v1.1 reagent (Applied Biosystems).
4. 2.5X sequencing buffer (Applied Biosystems).
5. Sephadex G50 DNA grade (Amersham Scientific, Piscataway, NJ).
6. 96-Well deep-well filter plates (Edge Biosystems, Gaithersburg, MD).
7. HiDi formamide (Applied Biosystems).
8. POP7 polymer (Applied Biosystems).
9. 3730 running buffer with EDTA (Applied Biosystems).

2.7. Equipment

1. Thermocycler.
2. Centrifuge.
3. Agarose gel electrophoresis apparatus and power supply.
4. WAVE Nucleic Acid Fragment Analysis System (Transgenomic).
5. Navigator™ software (Transgenomic).
6. Model 3730X1 DNA Analyzer (Applied Biosystems).
7. DNA Sequencing Analysis version 5.0 software (Applied Biosystems).
8. Chromas 2.0 software (www.Technelysium.com.au).

3. Methods

3.1. DNA Purification (Puregene Blood DNA Isolation Kit)

1. Put 9 mL whole blood into a 50-mL centrifuge tube with 27 mL Red Blood Cell Lysis Solution (Gentra Systems, Minneapolis, MN). Mix by inversion and let sit at room temperature for 5 min. Invert the sample and incubate at room temperature for another 5 min.
2. Centrifuge for 10 min at 4000 rpm (1500g). Remove the supernatant, being careful not to disturb the white cell pellet. Leave behind a small amount of liquid (about 200–400 μL).

3. Resuspend the white cell pellet by vortexing.
4. Add 9 mL Cell Lysis Solution (Gentra Systems) and mix with a pipet by drawing up and down multiple times to lyse the cells. If cell clumps are still visible, incubate at 56°C until solution is homogeneous.
5. Cool sample to room temperature.
6. Add 3 mL of Protein Precipitation Solution (Gentra Systems) to the cell lysate.
7. Vortex for 20 s.
8. Centrifuge at 4000 rpm (1500g) for 10 min, making sure that a brown protein pellet is formed. If pellet is not tight, repeat **step 7** and incubate on ice for 5 min and recentrifuge for 10 min.
9. Being careful not to disturb the protein pellet, pour the supernatant containing DNA into a 50-mL tube containing 9 mL of 100% isopropanol.
10. Mix by inversion about 50 times. Strands of precipitated DNA should appear.
11. Centrifuge at 4000 rpm (1500g) for 5 min. You should see a small white pellet of DNA.
12. Pour off the supernatant and gently stand the tube upside down on a paper towel to drain.
13. Add 5 mL of 70% ethanol and mix by inversion several times to clean the pellet.
14. Transfer the pellet to a 2-mL tube with a plastic pipet and centrifuge at 4000 rpm (1500g) for 5 min.
15. Carefully pipet off the alcohol, being sure not to disturb the pellet; it may be loose.
16. Allow the tube to sit at room temperature until the alcohol has evaporated, usually 10–15 min.
17. Depending on the size of the pellet, add a sufficient volume of DNA hydration solution (Gentra Systems) to obtain a concentration of 250 ng/μL.
18. Incubate at room temperature overnight on a rotating shaker.
19. Make a working aliquot of the DNA sample (25 ng/μL) by diluting 1/10 with DNA hydration solution (Gentra Systems).
10. Store DNA at 4°C or, for long-term storage, at –20 or –80°C.

3.2. Polymerase Chain Reaction

DNA amplification of all 60 coding region exons of the five LQTS-associated genes (*KCNQ1/KCNQ1* [exons 1–16], *KCNH2/HERG* [exons 1–15], *SCN5A* [exons 2–28], *KCNE1/MinK* [exon 4]), and *KCNE2/MiRP-1* [exon 2]) is conducted using a combination of previously described primer pairs and PCR conditions as well as primer pairs and PCR conditions for select amplicons developed in our laboratory (**Fig. 2**). Primer sequences and conditions are presented in **Tables 2–6**. Proper primer design is a critical step in this mutation detection process, as false-negatives secondary to poor primer design and possible allelic drop-out can occur (*see* **Fig. 3** and **Note 4**).

In general, PCR reactions are performed in 20-μL volumes using 50 ng of DNA, 16 pmol of each primer, 200 μM of each dNTP, 50 mM KCl, 10 mM Tris-HCl (pH 8.3), and either 1, 1.5, or 2 mM MgCl$_2$, and 1.0 U of Amplitaq

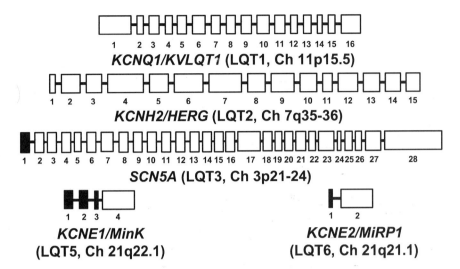

Fig. 2. Schematic representation of the long QT syndrome (LQTS)-associated channel gene structures. Depicted are the intron/exon structures for the LQTS-associated genes *KCNQ1*, *KCNH2*, *SCN5A*, *KCNE1*, and *KCNE2*. Protein-encoding exons ($n = 60$) are represented by white boxes, whereas black boxes represent noncoding exons. Intronic sequences are represented by the black line located between the boxes.

Gold (Applied Biosystems). Some PCR reactions require the addition of additives such as DMSO, glycerol, and/or formamide. PCR amplification is performed using a DNA Engine Tetrad thermal cylcer (MJ Research, Waltham, MA) with temperature cycling conditions individually optimized for each amplicon. As a result of consistently low PCR yield, some amplicons have been optimized using HotStarTaq DNA Polymerase (Qiagen) rather than Amplitaq Gold (Applied Biosystems).

1. Aliquot 2 µL of each DNA sample (25 ng/µL) into PCR plate or reaction tube. Remember to leave a well or tube open for a "No DNA" control.
2. Completely thaw and mix well by vortexing all components that have been frozen (5X PCR buffer and primers). *Do not* vortex DNA polymerase.
3. Following the recipe in **Table 1**, create a "master mix" by combining all PCR reagents, including polymerase, into a single microcentrifuge tube. Prepare enough mix to allow for pipetting error (i.e., make enough for 1 extra sample when performing PCR on 4 samples, enough for 10 extra samples when performing PCR on 96 samples). Some PCR amplicons have been optimized using slightly different conditions (i.e., different $MgCl_2$ concentrations, the use of additives such as DMSO, glycerol, and/or formamide, or HotStart Taq polymerase rather than Amplitaq Gold). *See* **Tables 2–6** for specific conditions for each amplicon.

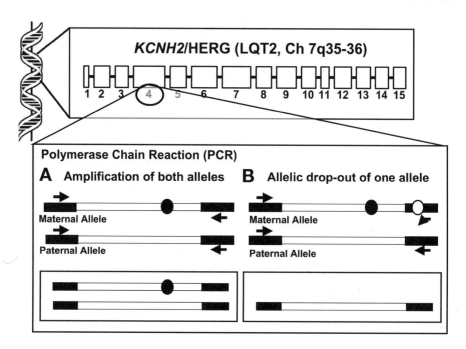

Fig. 3. Allelic drop-out: a possible mechanism explaining false-negative results. In order to understand how allelic drop-out can lead to false-negative results, we first need to explore the general design of how PCR is performed for mutation analysis using genomic DNA. By focusing on exon 4 of *KCNH2*, we can see how a PCR reaction is first designed in order to amplify both the maternal and parental alleles. By designing a forward and reverse primer complementary to flanking intronic DNA sequences, PCR products containing the desired exon can be generated. (**A**) If a mutation exists on one of the alleles as depicted here with a black circle, then PCR amplification of this sample would produce products containing the mutation that could be easily detected by most mutation detection platforms, such as denaturing high-performance liquid chromatography. (**B**) However, if a single-nucleotide polymorphism or SNP (white circle) located on the same allele as the mutation (black circle) and within the sequence complementary to the 3' end of the primer such that the primer annealing is disrupted, then amplification of that allele would not occur and the mutation would be missed. This in essence defines allelic drop-out.

4. Mix well by vortexing.
5. Centrifuge in a microcentrifuge for 5–10 s.
6. Aliquot 18 μL of the "master mix" to each 2-μL DNA sample.
7. Cover plate or tube with appropriate cover (plate cover or tube cap).
8. Place samples on thermal cycler and run the appropriate method. Annealing temperatures and cycling conditions vary by amplicon; *see* **Tables 2–6** for individual conditions.

Thermal cycling methods as presented in the PCR condition tables are as follows:

1. 94°C initial denaturation for 5 min, followed by 5 cycles of 94°C for 20 s, 64°C for 20 s, and 72°C for 30 s; then an additional 35 cycles of 94°C for 20 s, 62°C for 20 s, 72°C for 30 s, and a final extension of 72°C for 10 min.
2. 94°C initial denaturation for 15 min, followed by 35 cycles of 94°C for 30 s, 58°C for 30 s, 72°C for 30 s, and a final extension of 72°C for 10 min.
3. 94°C initial denaturation for 10 min, followed by 40 cycles of 94°C for 30 s, 55°C for 30 s, 72°C for 30 s, and a final extension of 72°C for 10 min.
4. 94°C initial denaturation for 10 min, followed by 40 cycles of 94°C for 30 s, 60°C for 30 s, 72°C for 30 s, and a final extension of 72°C for 10 min.

3.3. Agarose Check Gel (Optional)

Typically, we use 3% agarose check gels during initial optimization of newly designed PCR amplicons. Once PCR conditions are optimal, there is no need to perform a check gel prior to dHPLC analysis.

1. Put masking tape on the ends of the plastic gel form to obtain a tight seal. Depending on the apparatus, some gel forms will not require taping.
2. Place the desired comb in the gel form.
3. Dilute 10X TBE to a 1X concentration: 100 mL TBE to 900 mL 18 Ω-cm H_2O in large cylinder.
4. To prepare a 3% solution (3 g/100 mL TBE), measure out 3:1 high-resolution blend (HRB) agarose powder, place into a 500-mL flask, add 100 mL of 1X TBE, and "cork" with a paper towel.
5. Microwave for 30 s to dissolve.
6. Swirl to mix.
7. Microwave for another 30 s.
8. Carefully add 2.5 µL of ethidium bromide (carcinogen—USE GLOVES) to flask.
9. Swirl flask and pour into gel form.
10. Allow gel mix to cool and solidify for about 30 min at room temperature. Alternatively, the gel can be ready in 10 min if the solution is allowed to solidify at 4°C. Gels can be stored wrapped in a sealable plastic bag at 4°C until ready for use.
11. While the gel is setting, mix 10 µL of PCR product with 2 µL of 6X loading buffer.
12. Once the gel has set, gently remove the comb to avoid tearing the wells. Then remove the masking tape off the edges of the gel form.
13. Place the gel into the gel box oriented so that the samples run toward the positive (red) electrode.
14. Fill the gel box with 1X TBE, being sure that the entire gel is immersed in TBE.
15. Load 10 µL of DNA sizing ladder and PCR products into separate wells.
16. Place the lid on the gel box and connect the electrodes to the power supply.
17. Electrophorese at 96 V for about 1 h or until the orange dye front has moved approx 5 cm.
18. View the gel under UV light and take a picture if desired.

3.4. Denaturing High-Performance Liquid Chromatography

Mutational analysis is performed using dHPLC, utilizing a 3500HT DNA Fragment Analysis System (WAVE™), Transgenomic Inc., San Jose, CA). Five microliters of PCR product is loaded onto a preheated DNAsep HT cartridge (Transgenomic, cat. no. DNA-99-3710) and is eluted under partially denaturing conditions with a linear acetonitrile gradient composed of buffers A (0.1 *M* TEAA) and B (0.1 *M* TEAA and 25% ACN). A gradient of 5% buffer B per minute at a flow rate of 1.5 mL/min in WAVE 3500 HT rapid DNA mode allows mutation detection at temperatures optimized for each exon. Eluted DNA fragments are detected by UV absorption at a wavelength of 260 nm, and the resulting chromatograms are examined for abnormal elution profiles.

1. Check for proper column resolution prior to running samples using 5 μL of the Mutation Standard. This is a very important step (*see* **Note 5**).
2. Check for proper pressure. The pressure is normally between 900 and 1500 psi when the instrument is running 50% buffer A and 50% buffer B at 1.5 mL/min flow rate (*see* **Note 5**).
3. Check for proper buffer volume. A single plate of 96 samples will require a minimum of 500 mL of buffer A, 500 mL of buffer B, 300 mL of buffer C, and 200 mL of buffer D. Make the buffer and fill if necessary (*see* **Subheading 2.3.** and **Note 3**).
4. Check for air bubbles in buffer lines. Purge or prime lines if necessary.
5. PCR products are heated to 95°C for 5 min, and then allowed to cool to room temperature (*see* **Note 6**).
6. Create a project file/injection tray in Navigator software following manufacturer's instruction. Briefly, the injection tray will have all of the vital information, such as sample ID, vial numbers, sample injection volumes (5 μL), and method parameters (temperature and gradient), which the instrument will require to process the samples successfully (*see* **Tables 2–6** for dHPLC conditions).
7. Some PCR products will require more than one temperature to achieve full mutational analysis. If more than one temperature is needed, it is recommended that all PCR samples for the specific PCR fragment (exon) are analyzed at one temperature and that injections are then repeated for the second temperature (*see* **Note 7** and **Tables 2–6**).
8. Be sure to add an active wash method at the end every 96 samples on the injection tray. This is very important (*see* **Note 8**).
9. Once the plate of samples has been cooled to room temperature, place the plate on the chiller in the auto sampler.
10. After checking to be sure that the injection tray has been set up correctly, select Run Injections (green arrow) in Navigator software.
11. When running injections in high-throughput mode (1.5 mL/min flow rate, 2.5 min gradient), it will take approx 7–8 h to complete analysis of 96 samples for one temperature.

12. Once injections are complete, carefully analyze dHPLC chromatograms for abnormal profiles indicating the presence of heterzygote DNA variants using the analysis page and tools in Navigator software. For helpful tips on abnormal profile analysis, *see* **Note 9**.
13. Select samples for DNA sequencing. Remember to select a sample with a normal profile to use for sequence comparison with abnormal samples.
14. PCR samples for sequencing can be selected directly from the plate in which dHPLC was performed. If sample volume has been lost due to evaporation, rehydrating with 5 μL of 18 Ω-cm H_2O, when only a single 5-μL injection has been performed, can give sufficient PCR product for sequencing. If more than 5 μL of the PCR product has been injected for dHPLC analysis (i.e., two-temperature dHPLC), then samples to be sequenced will require re-PCR amplification.

3.5. Purification of PCR Template in Preparation for DNA Sequencing

1. To clean the PCR product for further analysis by automated DNA sequencing, 5 μL of PCR product is placed into a 0.2-mL reaction tube with 2 μL EXOSAP-IT (USB).
2. Cap the tube and using a thermal cycler, incubate the reaction mixture at 37°C for 15 min, then at 80°C for 15 min.
3. Store the reaction mixture at 4°C until ready to sequence.

3.6. Preparation of Sequencing Reaction Template

1. Take 1 μL of purified PCR product and place in an individual 0.2-mL PCR reaction tube.
2. Add 0.5 μL of forward primer (2 μ*M*).
3. Bring volume up to 6 μL with 18 Ω-cm H_2O and cap tube.

3.7. Sequencing Reaction

Steps 1–14 are performed by our sequencing core facility.

1. Place samples to be sequenced in a 96-well plate and centrifuge the plate at 1600*g* for 30 s.
2. 4 μL of Big Dye Terminator v1.1 reagent is added to all samples at a 1:2 ratio with 2.5X sequencing buffer.
3. The plate is covered and centrifuged again at 1600*g* for 30 s.
4. The plate is then put on the PCR machine and cycled 25 times at the following conditions: 96°C for 10 s, 50°C for 5 s, and 60°C for 4 min and then held at 4°C until ready to go to next step.
5. Remove plate from PCR machine and add 10 μL of 18 Ω-cm H_2O to each well in the plate.
6. Prepare a Sephadex G50 filter plate by adding 800 μL of a slurry of 700 mL 18 Ω-cm H_2O and 50 g DNA-grade Sephadex G50 to each well of a 96-well, deep-well filter plate.
7. Let plate sit for 2 h.

8. Centrifuge plate at 2400*g* for 2 min, blotting the bottom of the plate afterward to remove any excess water.
9. Transfer entire sample volume to the previously centrifuged 96-well filter plate containing DNA grade Sephadex G50.
10. Centrifuge filter plate once samples are added for 2 min at 2400*g*, collecting the purified sample into a new 96-well microtiter plate.
11. Dry the purified samples at 45°C for 55 min in a speedvac.
12. Resuspend samples with 10 µL HiDi formamide and shake plate at 2000 rpm for 3 min on a microplate shaker.
13. Place the plate onto the 3730xl DNA Analyzer and run as recommended by Applied Biosystems.
14. Analyze sequence data using DNA Sequencing Analysis v5.0.
15. Sequence chromatograms can be viewed and printed using Chromas 2.0 software.
16. Compare the normal sequence chromatogram with chromatograms from samples with abnormal dHPLC profiles to elucidate the underlying DNA change (*see* **Note 10**).

4. Notes

1. High-throughput laboratories will benefit from making a large quantity of 5X PCR buffer. We typically make 25 mL of 5X PCR buffer and aliquot 424 µL (enough buffer for a 106-sample "master mix") of buffer into separate 1.5-mL microtubes. Working aliquots of PCR buffer are stored at –20°C until ready for use. The remaining PCR reagents can be added to the micotube containing 424 µL of buffer when performing PCR for an entire rack of 96 samples.
2. Some PCR reactions have been optimized with the use of HotStart Taq DNA polymerase from Qiagen in place of Amplitaq Gold Polymerase. HotStart Taq requires HotStart Taq PCR buffer. This buffer contains 1.5 m*M* MgCl$_2$.
3. It is crucial that when making buffers A and B, that reagents are measured out precisely with a consistent effort. Failure to do so may affect the consistency of elution profile retention times and morphology between runs. Alternatively, premade buffers A, B, syringe wash (buffer C), and active wash (buffer D) can be purchased from Transgenomic.
4. Some possible explanations for genotype negative cases are incorrect LQTS diagnosis, mutations in novel genes waiting discovery, mutations located in unchartered territory (promoter regions or whole gene or exon deletions) of the known LQTS genes, or mutation detection failures such as technical or instrument misses, user misses, and PCR design failures such as allelic drop-out (*see* **Fig. 3**). Recently, our lab has identified LQTS-associated mutations in *KCNQ1* exon 15 and *KCNH2* exon 4 that had been previously missed as a result of allelic drop-out. Primer pairs to amplify these two exons have been redesigned and are reported here in **Tables 2** and **3**, respectively. Unfortunately, allelic drop-out can be difficult to detect unless the primer-disrupting SNP is present in a high enough frequency such that some samples will be homozygous for the primer disrupting SNP. This will result in nonamplification of those samples. If a set of samples

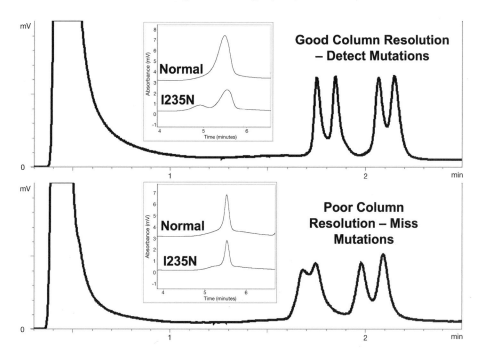

Fig. 4. The importance of good column resolution. Illustrated is the importance of good column resolution in mutation detection. (**A**) Shown is an example of perfect resolution of the Low Range Mutation Standard (Transgenomic) and in the inset is a denaturing high-performance liquid chromatography (dHPLC) chromatogram showing the easily detected abnormal elution profile for the *I235N-KCNQ1* mutation. (**B**) Depicted is an example of poor column resolution with the inset showing how the previously detectable *I235N-KCNQ1* can be easily missed when the column resolution is poor. This underscores the importance in maintaining proper column resolution and the need for mutation standard analysis as a part of the daily dHPLC regimen.

repeatedly do not amplify for a given PCR fragment yet work well for other fragments, then this may in fact represent allelic drop-out.

5. Proper column resolution is a must when it comes to effectively detecting mutations by dHPLC. Columns with poor resolving power may lead to mutation detection failure. This is illustrated in **Fig. 4**. If high pressure is observed in conjunction with poor resolution following injection of the mutation standard, it is advisable to change the in-line filter that immediately precedes the column. The column can be washed by running 100% Active Wash (75% acetonitrile) at a flow rate of 1.5 mL/min through the system with the oven set for 80°C for about 30 min. Re-equilibrate the column by running 50% buffer A and 50% buffer B at 1.5 mL/min flow rate for 1 h. Occasionally, if this extended wash fails to restore resolution, then washing in the same manner as just described with 18 Ω-cm H_2O

may improve the resolution of the column. To do this, simply substitute the "buffer A" bottle with a bottle of pure water and run the system with 100% "buffer A" (water). If column resolution is only slightly off and continues to persist, the oven may need to be recalibrated. Run the mutation standard at 0.5°C above and below the normal temperature in which the standard is normally run (i.e., 55.5°C, 56°C, and 56.5°C). If the resolution appears better at one of the new temperatures, then oven calibration according to the manufacture's guidelines may be necessary.

6. It has been recommended to denature the PCR products at 95°C and to re-anneal by allowing the samples to cool to room temperature prior to dHPLC. In our experience, we have found that mutation detection is not enhanced by doing this. Because denaturing and reannealing occur through out the process of thermal cycling, we simply take the samples directly from the thermal cycler to the dHPLC instrument. Samples can also be taken from the thermal cycler and stored at 4°C until ready for dHPLC.

7. In order to effectively detect all DNA changes within the PCR fragment, some fragments will require more than one temperature for complete analysis (*see* **Fig. 5**). Mutations may be missed if this rule is not adhered to diligently.

8. In order to maintain proper column resolution between runs, it is advisable to run an "active wash method" (100 % buffer D for 15 min, followed by 50% buffer A and 50% buffer B for 30 min all at a flow rate of 1.5 mL/min and at 80°C) after every 96 samples. The addition of this extended wash is extremely helpful in maintaining column resolution but is not a substitute for performing a mutation standard on a daily basis.

9. As a result of the highly reproducible nature of elution profiles for normal samples and samples with known mutations, reviewing dHPLC chromatograms consists of simply looking for profiles that are different. Such abnormal profiles may manifest with multiple peaks, shouldering of the normal profile, or widening of the normal profile. Normal profiles can show some level of natural variability in retention time and shape between samples. The best way to analyze abnormal profiles is to first visually determine what the range of natural variability is and then look for sample profiles that appear outside of that range. This is usually easily achieved because most samples analyzed will be "normal" for a given amplicon. Unique mutations tend to give reproducibly unique dHPLC profiles and can often be distinguished according to shape and retention times of the peaks. However, *be careful*, this does not always hold true and dHPLC should not be used for genotyping purposes. **Figure 6A** shows how two distinct heterozygous DNA variations can appear identical. This can be an extreme challenge when dealing with fragments that host common polymorphisms. Special care is needed to look for subtle differences either in retention time or peak morphology when trying to tease out abnormal profiles where the underlying DNA change is in fact a pathogenic mutation rather than the common polymorphism. Another challenge involves identification of those samples that have very subtle difference in the elution profile when compared with the normal profile (**Fig. 6B**). This may occur

A **Single Melt Temperature**

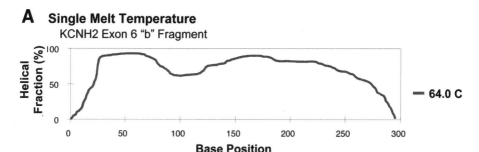

B **Multiple Melt Temperatures**

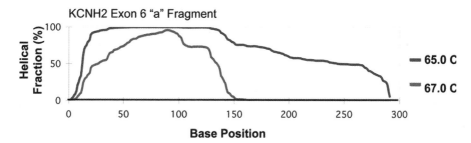

Fig. 5. Denaturing high-performance liquid chromatography (dHPLC) melt profiles as predicted by Navigator software. Mutations can be detected at base positions where the helical fraction (double stranded) is greater than 25% and less than 100%. (**A**) Depicted is the predicted melt profile for *KCNH2* exon 6b, which represents a single melt temperature fragment. A single temperature of 64°C can be used to detect mutations at any base position along the fragment as indicated by the red line. (**B**) Shown is the predicted melt profile for *KCNH2* exon 6a, which represents a multiple melt temperature fragment. Here, complete mutational analysis can only be achieved when the fragment is subject to dHPLC at both 65°C (base positions 140–300, red line) and 67°C (base position 1–145, blue line).

even when column resolution is optimal and emphasizes the importance of carefully examining all profiles. Again, taking special care to look for profiles that are outside of the normal range of variability can allow the user to detect these subtle profiles. Although the challenge of multiple mutations presenting as similar profiles and the challenge of mutations presenting as subtle abnormalities is the exception rather then the rule, mutation misses will occur if the investigator is not analyzing dHPLC chromatograms with these challenges in mind.

10. Some investigators will choose to use software tools to look for abnormal sequence changes. We simply print out the normal and suspected mutant color sequence chromatograms and look for sequence changes. Heterozygote single-nucleotide substitutions appear as double peaks as illustrated in **Fig. 7**, whereas

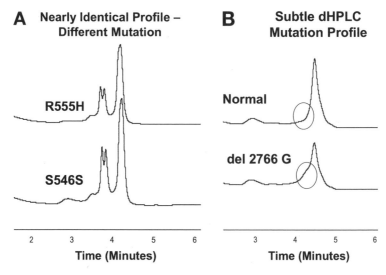

Fig. 6. Challenging denaturing high-performance liquid chromatography (dHPLC) chromatograms. Most often, DNA variants present with easily detectable, unique, and highly reproducible elution profiles; however, as shown in **A**, two different DNA variants can present with a nearly identical and indistinguishable elution profile. This makes genotyping by dHPLC difficult. The example shown here is from a "family screen" in which the family index case was known to be positive for the *R555H-KCNQ1* mutation. The uncle of the index case was found to have an identical dHPLC profile as the family mutation, yet when sequencing was performed, the uncle was shown to harbor a "silent" mutation and was negative for the R555H mutation. Genotyping by dHPLC alone would have lead to a misdiagnosis of long QT syndrome. Another challenge, as demonstrated in **B**, is that some mutant profiles can present as very subtle abnormalities even when column resolution is optimal. This is depicted by the circle.

heterozygote insertions and deletions appear as a series of double peaks immediately following the point of insertion or deletion as illustrated in **Fig. 8**. Mutation detection by sequencing relies vitally on clean chromatograms. If chromatograms contain a high level of "background noise," then sequencing should be repeated. Occasionally, sequencing artifact can be seen on chromatograms as double peaks. Careful scrutiny of the sequence chromatogram can prevent the misidentification of these artifacts as mutations. False-positive sequence artifacts can be distinguished from true heterozygote mutations by carefully looking at the "normal" peak. With a true heterozygote mutation, the chromatogram should show a diminution of the "normal" or "wild-type" peak as seen in **Fig. 7**; however if the "wild-type" peak does not reduce in size from what is seen on the "normal" chromatogram, then this most likely represents sequencing artifact. dHPLC has proven to be very effective in discovering samples con-

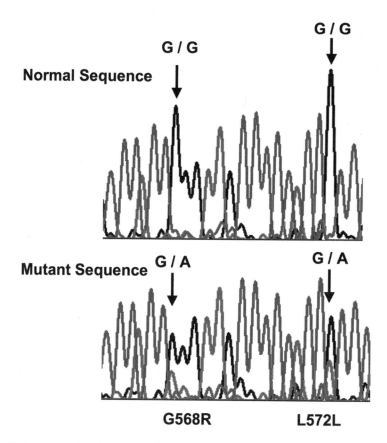

Fig. 7. An example of a sequencing chromatogram revealing a missense mutation and a synonymous single-nucleotide polymorphism. Depicted is an example of a normal and mutant sequence chromatogram revealing both the heterozygote *G568R-KVLQT1* pathogenic missense mutation and the heterozygote *L572L-KVLQT1* synonymous single nucleotide polymorphism, thus illustrating the need to thoroughly examine the entire chromatogram for possible nucleotide changes. Note the reduced size of the normal base (black peak = guanine), and the addition of a green peak (adenine) directly underneath it in the mutant sequence as compared with the normal sequence.

taining heterozygote DNA changes with very little to no false-positives. At least in our experience, whenever a sample presents with an obvious abnormal dHPLC elution profile, we always find the DNA change by sequencing. If sequencing fails to reveal a heterozygote DNA change in a sample with a clearly abnormal dHPLC profile, the mutation may be located near the primer sequence where resolution of the sequencing chromatogram is usually poor. Sequencing in the opposite direction (i.e., with the reverse primer) may aid in elucidating the

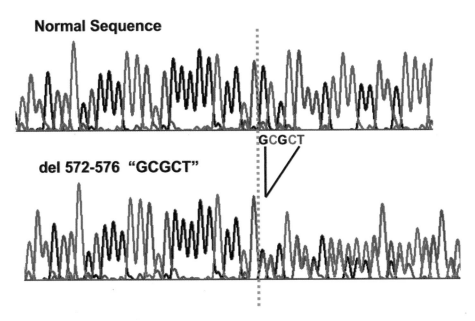

Normal Sequence

del 572-576 "GCGCT"

GCGCT

Fig. 8. An example of a sequencing chromatogram revealing a deletion mutation. Shown here are both a normal sequence chromatogram and mutant sequencing chromatogram revealing a heterozygote 5-bp deletion. The normal and mutant chromatograms appear to be identical until the point of deletion (gray dashed line). Note that after the point of deletion, some peaks are reduced and overlapped with an additional peak.

underlying DNA change. It is also advisable to confirm mutation detection by repeating PCR amplification and DNA sequencing.

Acknowledgments

The authors would like to extend there gratitude to Mr. Bruce Eckloff of the Mayo Clinic Sequencing Core for kindly supplying us with their sequencing protocol and to Ms. Maggie Karst for her expert advise in DNA isolation.

References

1. Curran, M. E., Splawski, I., Timothy, K. W., Vincent, G. M., Green, E. D., and Keating, M. T. (1995) A molecular basis for cardiac arrhythmia: HERG mutations cause long QT syndrome. *Cell* **80,** 795–803.
2. Wang, Q., Shen, J., Splawski, I., et al. (1995) SCN5A mutations associated with an inherited cardiac arrhythmia, long QT syndrome. *Cell* **80,** 805–811.
3. Splawski, I., Shen, J., Timothy, K. W., et al. (2000) Spectrum of mutations in long-QT syndrome genes. KVLQT1, HERG, SCN5A, KCNE1, and KCNE2. *Circulation* **102,** 1178–1185.

4. Tester, D. J., Will, M. L., Haglund, C. M., and Ackerman, M. J. (2005) Compendium of cardiac channel mutations in 541 consecutive unrelated patients referred for long QT syndrome genetic testing. *Heart Rhythm* **2,** 507–517.

5. Keating, M. T. and Sanguinetti, M. C. (2001) Molecular and cellular mechanisms of cardiac arrhythmias. *Cell* **104,** 569–580.

6. Ackerman, M. J. (2004) Cardiac channelopathies: it's in the genes. *Nature Medicine* **10,** 463–464.

7. Ning, L., Moss, A., Zareba, W., et al. (2003) Novel compound heterozygous mutations in the KCNQ1 gene associated with autosomal recessive long QT syndrome (Jervell and Lange-Nielsen syndrome). *Genetic Testing* **7,** 249–253.

8. Spiegelman, J. I., Mindrinos, M. N., and Oefner, P. J. (2000) High-accuracy DNA sequence variation screening by DHPLC. *BioTechniques* **29,** 1084–1092.

9. Ackerman, M. J., Splawski, I., Makielski, J. C., et al. (2004) Spectrum and prevalence of cardiac sodium channel variants among black, white, Asian, and Hispanic individuals: implications for arrhythmogenic susceptibility and Brugada/long QT syndrome genetic testing. *Heart Rhythm* **1,** 600–607.

10. Ackerman, M. J., Tester, D. J., Jones, G., Will, M. K., Burrow, C. R., and Curran, M. (2003) Ethnic differences in cardiac potassium channel variants: implications for genetic susceptibility to sudden cardiac death and genetic testing for congenital long QT syndrome. *Mayo Clinic Proceedings* **78,** 1479–1487.

11. Splawski, I., Shen, J., Timothy, K. W., Vincent, G. M., Lehmann, M. H., and Keating, M. T. (1998) Genomic structure of three long QT syndrome genes: KVLQT1, HERG, and KCNE1. *Genomics* **51,** 86–97.

12. Wang, Q., Li, Z., Shen, J., and Keating, M. T. (1996) Genomic organization of the human SCN5A gene encoding the cardiac sodium channel. *Genomics* **34,** 9–16.

13. Abbott, G. W., Sesti, F., Splawski, I., et al. (1999) MiRP1 forms IKr potassium channels with HERG and is associated with cardiac arrhythmia. *Cell* **97,** 175–187.

14. Itoh, T., Tanaka, T., Nagai, R., et al. (1998) Genomic organization and mutational

14

High-Throughput Single-Nucleotide Polymorphisms Genotyping

Taqman Assay and Pyrosequencing Assay

Gong-Qing Shen, Albert Luo, and Qing K. Wang

Summary

Single-nucleotide polymorphisms (SNPs) are DNA sequence variations that occur at a single base in the genome sequence. SNPs are valuable markers for identifying genes responsible for susceptibility to common diseases, and in some cases, they are the causes of human diseases. A genetic study of a complex disease usually involves a case–control association study that requires genotyping of a large number of SNPs in hundreds of patients (cases) and matched controls. A significant difference of the allele frequency or genotypic frequency of a SNP between the two populations is considered to be the evidence for the association between the SNP and disease. A key to a fast and effective case–control association study requires high-throughput genotyping of SNPs. Two assays—the TaqMan SNP genotyping assay and the pyrosequencing assay—have been developed for this purpose and proven to be particularly useful. Here, we present the operative protocol, clarify the key technical issues, and highlight certain cautionary notes for high throughput SNP genotyping using TaqMan and pyrosequencing assays.

Key Words: Genotyping; genetics of complex disease; case–control association study; single-nucleotide polymorphism; SNP; genetic variation; polymorphism; susceptibility gene.

1. Introduction

A single-nucleotide polymorphism (SNP) is a variation in a DNA base pair in which one coding letter of the four nucleotides (either A, G, T, or C) is substituted by a different letter. SNPs can be used as polymorphic markers in linkage analysis to map the chromosomal location of a disease or a complex genetic trait, and in some cases, they represent mutations that are causative to

From: *Methods in Molecular Medicine, Vol. 128: Cardiovascular Disease; Methods and Protocols; Volume 1*
Edited by: Q. Wang © Humana Press Inc., Totowa, NJ

the disease *(1,2)*. SNPs are the most abundant type of human genetic variations *(3,4)*. More than 3 million SNPs are thought to exist in the human genome, and their typical frequency is estimated to be 1–2 per 1000 bp *(5)*. Many SNPs are polymorphisms for which the rare allele is present at or above 1% frequency in the population *(6)*. Because SNPs occur frequently throughout the genome, tend to be relatively stable genetically, and can be genotyped quite easily, they serve as an excellent tool for performing a whole-genome association study to identify a susceptibility gene for a common complex disease or trait *(7)*. Furthermore, SNPs have already gained wide acceptance as genetic markers for use in linkage and association studies and have been used for large-scale case–control association studies in coronary artery disease, myocardial infarction, stroke, hypertension, and other cardiovascular diseases *(8–16)*.

The rapidly increasing utility of SNP genotyping has recently prompted the question of the number of SNPs needed to identify genes for complex disease traits. It has been estimated that approx 50,000–100,000 SNPs would be needed for a whole-genome association study *(17)*. Even for large-scale case–control association studies, thousands to millions of SNP genotypes must be generated quickly. For these studies, high-throughput genotyping platforms are required. In the last several years, SNP genotyping technology has rapidly evolved with the development of fast and novel methods *(18–24)*. In this chapter, we focus on the methods of the advanced and widely used TaqMan SNP genotyping assay using ABI Prism 7900HT Sequence Detection System (Applied Biosystems, Foster City, CA) *(25–27)* and the pyrosequencing assay using Pyrosequencing PSQ HS 96 (Pyrosequencing AB, Uppsala, Sweden) *(28–30)*. We will discuss the operative protocol, clarify some technical issues, and highlight several cautionary notes involved in high throughput SNP genotyping.

The TaqMan assay or the 5' nuclease allelic discrimination assay requires the forward PCR primer, the reverse primer, and two differently labeled TaqMan minor groove binder (MGB) probes in which the bi-allelic SNP is designed in the middle third of the probe. Each allele-specific MGB probe is labeled with a fluorescent reporter dye, either a FAM or VIC reporter molecule, and is attached with a fluorescence quencher Q. For the intact MGB probe, the reporter dye is quenched. During PCR, the 5' nuclease activity of Taq DNA polymerase cleaves the reporter dye (F or V) from an MGB probe that is completely hybridized to the DNA strand. When separated from quencher Q, the reporter dye fluoresces. However, if a single-point mismatch is present between the probe and target DNA strand as a result of an SNP, the binding of the probe to DNA is destabilized during strand displacement in PCR, which will reduce the efficiency of probe cleavage and quenching of the fluorescent reporter dye. Therefore, an increase in either FAM or VIC dye fluorescence indicates homozygosity for FAM- or VIC-specific alleles (1:1 and 2:2), and an increase in both dyes indicates heterozygosity (1:2). The ABI 7900HT system can distinguish and quantify the two colors (FAM or VIC), and genotypes can be generated for many samples in a few minutes.

The pyrosequencing assay or Pyrosequencing PSQ HS 96 is a molecular genetic technique for quick and exact analysis of short-length, direct DNA sequences. It is based on the principle of sequencing by synthesis. After PCR amplification of a specific region with an SNP to be genotyped, the PCR product is incubated with four enzymes (DNA polymerase, ATP sulfurylase, luciferase, and apyrase) and the two substrates (adenosine 5' phosphosulfate [APS] and luciferin). The sequencing primer is then added, which hybridizes to single-strand DNA (PCR product) and starts the cascade reactions. Starting from the primer, DNA polymerase catalyzes the incorporation of the first of four deoxynucleotide triphosphates (dNTPs) into the DNA strand and releases the pyrophosphate (PPi). ATP sulfurylase quantitatively converts both APS and PPi to ATP. The luciferase converts the ATP to visible light that is seen as a peak. Apyrase is a nucleotide-degrading enzyme, and it degrades unincorporated dNTP and excess ATP in the reaction. If the nucleotide is incorporated, a light signal is generated, and the complementary DNA base is registered and the DNA strand is built up. A peak referring to the sequence of DNA base is shown on the results tab. The height of each peak is proportional to the number of nucleotides incorporated. If the added nucleotide does not find complementation to the next DNA base in the template, light is not generated and it does not show any peak on the results tab. Up to 96 samples can be prepared and analyzed at the same time, and the total time needed for the run is only 1 h.

2. Materials

2.1. Preparation of High-Quality DNA Samples Using the DNA Isolation Kit for Mammalian Blood (Roche)

1. Transfer 10 mL of whole blood stored in EDTA or heparin to a sterile 50-mL centrifuge tube and add 30 mL of red blood cell lysis buffer.
2. Gently shake for 10 min, and centrifuge the tube at 900g for 10 min at 4°C.
3. Remove supernatant (blood waste), add 5 mL white blood cell lysis buffer, vortex thoroughly, and incubate for 30 min at 65°C.
4. Add 2.6 mL protein precipitation solution, vortex thoroughly, and centrifuge the sample at 12,000g for 25 min at 4°C (*see* **Note 1**).
5. Transfer the supernatant into a new sterile 50-mL centrifuge tube, add 2 vol of room-temperature 100% ethanol, and gently mix by inversion until DNA strands precipitate out of solution.
6. Carefully remove the DNA strands from the 100% ethanol using a pipet tip or toothpick and transfer to a new 1.5-mL microcentrifuge tube containing 1 mL cold 70% ethanol, gently mix the sample two to three times, and centrifuge the tube at 12,000g for 10 min at 4°C.

7. Discard the supernatant, and air-dry the DNA pellet for 3–4 h.
8. Add 1 mL of TE buffer (pH 8.0), vortex, and incubate at 65°C for 2 h.
9. Measure the concentration of DNA using a spectrophotometer. Store the DNA samples in a 4°C refrigerator or an –80°C freezer until use.

2.2. Preparation of 384-Well DNA Plate

Although 96-well plates can be used, 384-well reaction plates are preferred for running high-throughput SNP genotyping because they not only facilitate the screening of more samples simultaneously but also save costs on reagents and other materials. Because of their narrow, dense wells, DNA samples are best loaded into 384-well plates using the Hydra II microdispenser (**Fig. 1**). The Hydra II microdispenser is an instrument providing high-speed, repetitive aspirating and dispensing of microliter and nanoliter volumes into microplates and other receptacles. The machine can handle up to 384 channels of sample dispensing at the same time, and performs aspiration, dispensing, washing, and emptying functions.

1. Dilute DNA to a concentration of 12.5 ng/µL.
2. Prepare 384-well reaction plates (Applied Biosystems).
3. Press the **Power Switch** on the Hydra II microdispenser to **ON**.
4. Use the buttons on the front of the microdispenser to edit files (the file number from 1 to 16) including the settings for the operations of Dispense Aspirate, Empty, and Wash. Then use the same buttons to execute those operations.
5. Press **Wash** to start the washing operation. The syringe needles should be washed five times before aspiration.
6. Press **Aspr** to start the aspirate operation.
7. Press **Disp** to start dispense operation.
8. Set the tray table/stage height.
   a. Click **Page** so the Dispense screen appears on the display.
   b. From the **Dispense** screen, press **Edit** until the **Table** is on the top line of the screen.
   c. Press **Up** (slowly) to move the table/stage up until the needle tips are just touching the bottom of the wells in the plate (*see* **Note 2**). If the plate lifts easily, the tips are not at near bottom. Keep pressing **Up** (slowly) until you cannot lift the plate.
9. Set the file parameters.
   a. From the **Ready Mode** screen, press **Up** until **File 1** appears in the screen.
   b. Click **Page**, and the **Dispense** screen should then be in the display.
   c. From the **Dispense** screen, press **Edit** until **Vol** is on the top line of the screen. Set **Vol** to **10.0/40.0/70.0/120.0** by pressing **Up** or **Down**.
   d. Press **Edit** until **Table** is on the top line of the screen. Set **Table** to **3500** by pressing **Up** or **Down**.
   e. Press **Edit** until **Speed** is on the top line of the screen. Set **Speed** to **5** by pressing **Up** or **Down**.

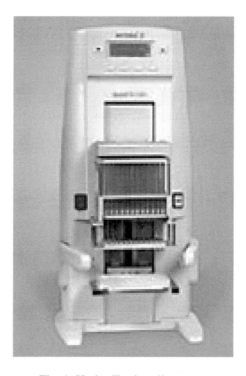

Fig. 1. Hydra II microdispenser.

f. Click **Page**, and the **Aspirate** screen should then be in the display.
g. From the **Aspirate** screen, press **Edit** until **Prime** is on the top line of the screen. Set **Prime** to **ON** by pressing **Up** or **Down**.
h. Press **Edit** until **Vol** is on the top line of the screen. Set **Vol** to **50.0/170.0/290.0/500.0** by pressing **Up** or **Down**.
i. Press **Edit** until **Air** is on the top line of the screen. Set **Air** to **0** by pressing **Up** or **Down**.
j. Press **Edit** until **Table** is on the top line of the screen. Set **Table** to **2700** by pressing **Up** or **Down**.
k. Press **Edit** until **Speed** is on the top line of the screen. Set **Speed** to **5** by pressing **Up** or **Down**.
l. Click **Page**, and the **Empty** screen should then be on the display.
m. From the **Empty** screen, press **Edit** until **Table** is on the top line of the screen. Set **Table** to **2500** by pressing **Up** or **Down**.
n. Press **Edit** until **Speed** is on the top line of the screen. Set **Speed** to **5** by pressing **Up** or **Down**.
o. Click **Page**, and the **Wash** screen should then be in the display.
p. From the **Wash** screen, press **Edit** until **Wash** is on the top line of the screen. Set **Wash** to **3** by pressing **Up** or **Down**.

q. Press **Edit** until **Vol** is on the top line of the screen. Set **Vol** to **60.0/190.0/340.0/560.0** by pressing **Up** or **Down**.

r. Press **Edit** until **Table** is on the top line of the screen. Set **Table** to **6500** by pressing **Up** or **Down**.

s. Press **Edit** until **Speed** is on the top line of the screen. Set **Speed** to **5** by pressing **Up** or **Down**.

t. Click **Page**, and the display should then be return to the **Ready Mode** screen.

10. Start to run a procedure.

a. Place a sample plate on the tray table/stage, then press **Aspr.**, the syringes aspirate the total amount of volumes of reagents.

b. Remove the plate from the table/stage.

c. Place the first receiving plate on the table/stage.

d. Press **Disp** on the right side of the microdispenser. The volume of the reagent is dispensed into the plate.

e. Remove the plate from the table/stage, place the next receiving plate until the last receiving plate is completed.

f. Press **Empty**.

g. Press **Wash** to wash the syringes.

2.3. Primer and Probe Design for ABI Prism 7900HT Sequence Detection System

High-throughput genotyping of SNPs using ABI Prism 7900HT Sequence Detection System (**Fig. 2**) employs the 5' nuclease allelic discrimination assay *(31–35)*. The assay includes the forward target-specific PCR primer, the reverse primer, and the TaqMan MGB probes labeled with two special dyes—FAM and VIC (*see* **Note 3**). Both Assays-on-Demand and Assays-by-Design services are offered by Applied Biosystems, Inc.

2.3.1. Assays-on-Demand (see **Note 4**)

1. Go to: http://www.appliedbiosystems.com.
2. Register and log in.
3. Enter TaqMan SNP genotyping assays and target gene name.
4. Choose SNP assay ID and add product to "Shopping Basket."
5. Proceed to checkout.

2.3.2. Assays-by-Design (see **Note 5**)

1. Choose the DNA target sequence. The sequence length is usually between 300 and 600 bases in the 5' to 3' orientation.
2. Designate the target SNP site with square brackets, e.g., ACCA[G/A]CTAG.
3. Provide a suitable name for the sequence record.
4. Submit the order by e-mail or regular mail to Applied Biosystems.

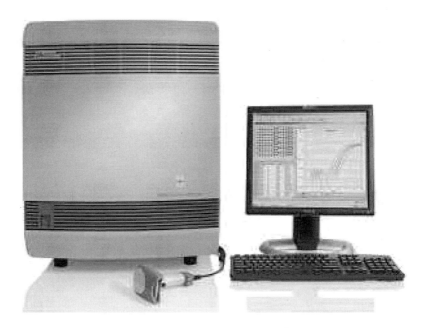

Fig. 2. ABI Prism 7900HT Sequence Detection System.

2.3.3. Primer and Probe Design Using Primer Express Software

Primer and probe can also be designed using Primer Express 2.0 Software.

1. Design a TaqMan probe using the following guidelines:
   a. Keep the G-C content in the 20 to 80% range.
   b. Select the strand that gives the probe more Cs than Gs.
   c. Do not put G on the 5' end.
   d. Avoid runs of an identical nucleotide. This is especially true for guanine, where runs of four or more Gs should be avoided.
   e. The melting temperature should be 65–67°C.
   f. Position the polymorphic site approximately in the middle third of the sequence.
   g. Adjust the probe lengths so that both probes have the same temperature.
2. Design a TaqMan primer using the following guidelines:
   a. Keep the G-C content in the 30 to 80% range.
   b. Avoid runs of an identical nucleotide. This is especially true for guanine, where runs of four or more Gs should be avoided.
   c. The melting temperature should be 58–60°C.
   d. The five nucleotides at the 3' end should have no more than two G and/or C bases.

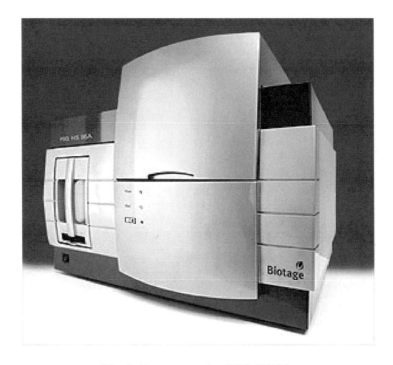

Fig. 3. Pyrosequencing PSQ HS 96.

e. Place the forward and reverse primers as close as possible to the probe without overlapping the probe.

2.4. PCR and Sequencing Primer Design for Pyrosequencing PSQ HS 96

Pyrosequencing PSQ HS 96 (**Fig. 3**) is a highly sensitive, quantitative genetic analysis system that can be used for SNP genotyping. Pyrosequencing assay typically offers greater than 99% reproducibility and accuracy (*see* **Note 6**).

2.4.1. PCR Primer Design

1. The length of PCR product should be <200 bp and the primer length of is approx 18–24 bases.
2. The calculated annealing temperature should be 62–65°C.
3. There should be no loops with a more than 6-bp match in the 3' end.
4. Biotin-label one of the primers for immobilization to magnetic or sepharose beads.
5. Purify the biotinylated primer using high-performance liquid chromatography (HPLC) (*see* **Note 7**).

2.4.2. Sequencing Primer Design

1. The length of PCR product should be <200 bp, and the length of primer approx 18–24 bases.

2. Annealing temperature should be around 50°C.
3. There should be no loops with more than a 6-bp match in the 3' end.
4. The primer should be flexible within five bases from the SNP for the primer position.

2.5. PCR Reaction for ABI Prism 7900HT Sequence Detection System

2.5.1. Assays-on-Demand

TaqMan Universal PCR Master Mix (2X)	2.5 μL
TaqMan MGB SNP genotyping assay mix (20X)	0.25 μL
DNA samples (12.5 ng/mL)	2 μL
Water	0.25 μL
Total	5 μL

2.5.2. Assays-by-Design

TaqMan Universal PCR Master Mix (2X)	2.5 μL
SNP genotyping assay mix (40X)	0.125 μL
DNA samples (12.5 ng/mL)	2 μL
Water	0.375 μL
Total	5 μL

2.6. PCR Reaction for Pyrosequencing PSQ HS 96

DNA samples (12.5 ng/mL)	1 μL
Forward primer (0.5 mM)	1 μL
Reverse primer (0.5 mM)	1 μL
10X dNTP (2.5 mM)	2.5 μL
10X PCR Gold buffer	2.5 μL
MgCl$_2$ solution (25 mM)	1.25 μL
AmpliTaq Gold (5 U/μL)	0.2 μL
Water	15.5 μL
Total volume	25 μL

3. Methods

3.1. TaqMan Assay

3.1.1. PCR

The PCR mixture is assembled as described previously, and PCR is carried out in GeneAmp PCR System 9700.

1. Press the **Power Switch** on the front of machine to the **ON** position.
2. From the **Main menu** screen, press **User** to display the Select **User Name** screen. Press **New** to add a new name to the list.
3. From the **User Name** screen, enter a unique name up to six characters in length.
4. Press **Accept** to accept a name.
5. From the **Main menu** screen, press **User** to display the Select **User Name** screen.

6. From the **User Name** screen, select the name that you just type it, and then click **Accept**.
7. From the **Main menu** screen, press **Edit** to display the Select **View** screen.
8. Enter time and temperature, and then click **Start**. The time and temperature of PCR for TaqMan SNP genotyping assay are as follows: one cycle of denaturation at 95°C for 10 min, 40 cycles of denaturation at 95°C for 15 s, and annealing at 60°C for 60 s; soak at 4°C until use.
9. From the **Select Method Options** screen, enter a value reaction for 5 µL, and then click **Start** again.

3.1.2. Genotyping

Genotyping or allele-calling is carried out in the ABI Prism 7900HT Genetic Detection System.

1. Turn **ON** the monitor and computer first, and then turn **ON** the 7900HT instrument. If the instrument is active normally, the solid green light on the front of the instrument is **ON**.
2. Select **Start > Programs > Applied Biosystems > SDS 2.1 > SDS 2.1**, or double-click the **SDS 2.1** icon on the monitor of computer.
3. Select **File > New**.
4. Configure the **New Document** dialog box with the following settings:

   - In the **Assay** drop-down list, select **Allelic Discrimination**.
   - In the **Container** drop-down list, select **384 Wells Clear Plate**.
   - In the **Template** drop-down list, select **Blank Template**.

5. Click **OK**.
6. From the SDS 2.1 software, select **Tools > Detector Manager**.
7. From the **Detector Manager** dialog box, select **New**.
8. From the **Add Detector** dialog box, click the **Name** field, and enter a unique name for the detector; in the **Reporter** drop-down list, select **FAM**, then click **OK** to save the detector and return to the **Detector Manager** dialog box.
9. From the **Detector Manager** dialog box, select **New** again.
10. From the **Add Detector** dialog box, click the **Name** field, and enter a different name for the detector; in the **Reporter** drop-down list, select **VIC**, then click **OK** and return to the **Detector Manager** dialog box.
11. Pressing the "Ctrl" key on the keyboard, select the detectors you want and highlight them, then click **Create Marker**.
12. From **Marker Editor**, click the **Name** field, type a new name, and then click **OK**.
13. From the **Detector Manager** dialog box, click **Done**.
14. From the SDS 2.1 software, select **Tools > Marker Manager**.
15. From the **Marker Manager** dialog box, search the name you just typed and highlight it.
16. Click **Copy To Plate Document**.

17. From **Copy Markers To Plate** dialog box, to make sure the name you wanted is correct, then click **OK**.
18. From the **Marker Manager** dialog box, click **Done**.
19. From the **Allelic Discrimination** dialog box, use the Ctrl and Shift keys and select the wells of the plate grid.
20. Click the **Use** check box of the marker you want to add to the selected wells.
21. From the **Allelic Discrimination** dialog box, click the **Instrument**.
22. From the **Plate Read** dialog box, first click **Connect**, and then click **Open/Close**. The instrument tray rotates to the OUT position. Transfer the PCR reaction plate from GeneAmp PCR System 9700 to the tray. Click **Open/Close** again. The instrument tray rotates to the IN position.
23. Click **Post Read**.
24. When running finishes, click **OK**.

3.1.3. The Data Analyses

1. Click the **Results** tab.
2. Click the lasso tool.
3. Select the sample cluster.
4. From the **Call** drop-down list, select **Allele X** call.
5. Select the other sample cluster, call them **Allele Y** or **Both**.
6. From the **File** menu, select **Print Report** (**Fig. 4**).

3.2. Pyrosequencing Assay

3.2.1. PCR

The PCR mixture is assembled as described previously and the PCR reaction is carried out in GeneAmp PCR System 9700. The procedure is as described for the TaqMan assay, except that the PCR amplification profile includes one cycle of denaturation at 95°C for 5 min, 40 cycles of denaturation at 94°C for 30 s, annealing at 60°C for 45 s and extension at 72°C for 60 s, an extension cycle at 72°C for 5 min, and a soak at 4°C until use. Check the PCR products on 1% agarose gel.

3.2.2. Genotyping

The following is a step-by-step procedure for operating the Pyrosequencing PSQ HS 96 system.

1. Order reagent kits and consumables (Pyro Gold, Biotage Inc., Uppsala, Sweden).
2. Add 25 μL of 2X binding buffer and 20 μL of Dynabeads into 25 μL of PCR products (*see* **Subheading 3.2.1.**).
3. Incubate at 65°C for 15 min, agitating constantly to keep the beads dispersed.
4. Add 100 μL of anneal buffer and 50 μL of washing buffer to wash the samples.
5. Add 200 μL of SNP reagent (SNP reagent kit) and 45 μL of sequencing primer to each well.

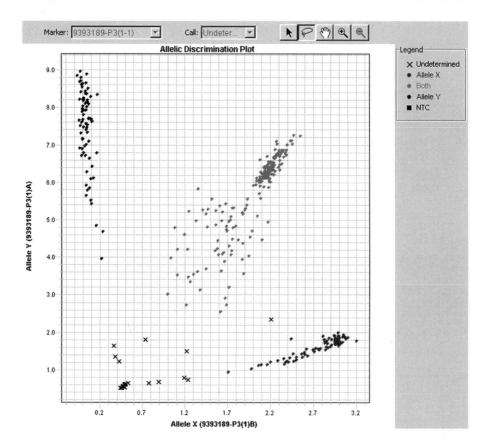

Fig. 4. The SDS 2.1 software can create a graph showing the results of allelic discrimination (allele calling). The clustering of these data points can vary along the horizontal axis (Allele X homozygote), vertical axis (Allele Y homozygote), and diagonal (Allele X/Allele Y heterozygote). A sample with a call indicated by the red spot represents homozygosity for one allele of a SNP (XX), the blue spot represents homozygosity for the other allele (YY), and a green spot is heterozygous (X/Y).

6. Place the 96-well sample plate into Pyrosequencing PSQ HS 96 system.
7. Assign each sample a genotype with simple color codes to indicate the confidence levels for each scored genotype.
8. Automatically score the results of each sample (**Fig. 5**).

4. Notes

1. Vortex continuously for 25 s. This is necessary for effective removal of protein from the sample.
2. It is crucial to know how to set the tray table/stage heights, so that neither operator nor instrument is at risk for damages when the microdispenser is operating. In

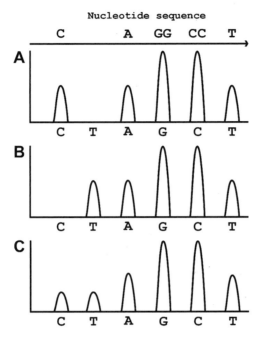

Fig. 5. Schematic drawing of the pyrosequencing results for SNP genotyping. The nucleotide sequence is [C/T]AGGCCT. The figure shows three different genotypes. (**A**) Homozygous CC alleles. (**B**) Homozygous TT alleles. (**C**) Heterozygous C/T alleles.

general, do not allow the needles to contact the bottom of any plate, tube, reservoir, tray, or wash basin. Use the fingertips to gently tilt the front edge of the plate up off of the table/stage and toward the needle tips.

3. The primers are used to amplify the SNP of interest, and the probes to detect the two different alleles.

4. Assays-on-Demand is a service of Applied Biosystems that provides ready-made SNP genotyping assays. The customer must submit sequence information and allele frequency. Assays are immediately available for over 100,000 SNPs in the ABI database.

5. If the SNP of interest is not in the database, ABI provides the Assays-by-Design service as an alternative. Assays-by-Design is a service that designs, synthesizes, formulates, and delivers analytically quality-controlled probe sets for SNP genotyping assays based on specific information submitted by the customer.

6. The pyrosequencing assay requires two different primers—PCR primer and sequencing primer. The PCR primers include forward and reverse primers, and the sequencing primer is the forward primer only. One of the PCR primers (usually using forward primer) is biotin-labeled for immobilization to magnetic or sepharose beads. The other PCR primer is unlabeled. The sequencing primer is also unlabeled.

7. Because free molecules of biotin will compete with the biotinylated PCR product for binding to streptavidin, purification of the biotinylated primer by HPLC is required.

Acknowledgments

This work was supported by the National Institutes of Health (NIH) grants R01 HL65630, R01 HL66251, P50 HL77107, and an American Heart Association Established Investigator award (to Q.W.).

References

1. Collins, F. S., Guyer, M. S., and Chakravarti, A. (1997) Variations on a theme: cataloging human DNA sequence variation. *Science* **278,** 1580–1581.
2. Sander, C. (2000) Genomic medicine and the future of health care. *Science* **287,** 1977–1978.
3. Brookes, A. J. (1999) The essence of SNPs. *Gene* **234,** 177–186.
4. Suh, Y. and Vijg, J. (2005) SNP discovery in associating genetic variation with human disease phenotypes. *Mutat. Res.* **573,** 41–53.
5. Kwok, P. Y. and Gu, Z. (1999) Single nucleotide polymorphism libraries: why and how are we building them? *Mol. Med. Today* **5,** 538–543.
6. Buetow, K. H., Edmondson, M. N., and Cassidy, A. B. (1999) Reliable identification of large numbers of candidate SNPs from public EST data. *Nat. Genet.* **21,** 323–325.
7. Picoult-Newberg, L., Ideker, T. E., Pohl, M. G., et al. (1999) Mining SNPs from EST databases. *Genome Res.* **9,** 167–174.
8. Topol, E. J., McCarthy, J., Gabriel, S., et al. (2001) Single nucleotide polymorphisms in multiple novel thrombospondin genes may be associated with familial premature myocardial infarction. *Circulation* **104,** 2641–2644.
9. Shen, G. Q., Archacki, S., and Wang, Q. (2004) The molecular genetics of coronary artery disease and myocardial infarction. *Acute Coronary Syndromes* **6,** 129–141.
10. Wang, Q. (2005) Advances in the genetic basis of coronary artery disease. *Curr. Atheroscler. Rep.* **7,** 235–241.
11. Gretarsdottir, S., Thorleifsson, G., Reynisdottir, S. T., et al. (2003) The gene encoding phosphodiesterase 4D confers risk of ischemic stroke. *Nat. Genet.* **35,** 131–138.
12. Ozaki, K., Ohnishi, Y., Iida, A., et al. (2002) Functional SNPs in the lymphotoxin-α gene that are associated with susceptibility to myocardial infarction. *Nat. Genet.* **32,** 650–654.
13. Garcia, E. C., Gonzalez, P., Castro, M. G., et al. (2003) Association between genetic variation in the Y chromosome and hypertension in myocardial infarction patients. *Am. J. Med. Genet.* **122,** 234–237.
14. Spiecker, M., Darius, H., Hankeln, T., et al. (2004) Risk of coronary artery disease associated with polymorphism of the cytochrome P450 epoxygenase CYP2J2. *Circulation* **110,** 2132–2136.

15. Pajukanta, P., Lilja, H. E., Sinsheimer, J. S., et al. (2004) Familial combined hyperlipidemia is associated with upstream transcription factor 1 (USF1). *Nat. Genet.* **36,** 371–376.
16. Helgadottir, A., Manolescu, A., Thorleifsson, G., et al. (2004) The gene encoding 5-lipoxygenase activating protein confers risk of myocardial infarction and stroke. *Nat. Genet.* **36,** 233–239.
17. Eric, L. (2001) Application of SNP technologies in medicine: lessons learned and future challenges. *Genome Res.* **11,** 927–929.
18. Weiss, K. M. and Terwilliger, J. D. (2000) How many disease does it take to map a gene with SNPs? *Nat. Genet.* **26,** 151–157.
19. Jenkins, S. and Gibson, N. (2002) High-throughput SNP genotyping. *Comp. Funct. Genom.* **3,** 57–66.
20. Tsuchihashi, Z. and Dracopoli, N. C. (2002) Progress in high throughput SNP genotyping methods. *Pharmacogenomics J.* **2,** 103–110.
21. Dearlove, A. M. (2002) High throughput genotyping technologies. *Brief Funct. Genomic Proteomic.* **1,** 139–150.
22. Wolford, J. K., Blunt, D., Ballecer, C., and Prochazka, M. (2000) High-throughput SNP detection by using DNA pooling and denaturing high performance liquid chromatography (DHPLC). *Hum. Genet.* **107,** 483–487.
23. Ohnishi, Y. (2002) A high-throughput SNP typing system for genome-wide association studies. *Gan To Kagaku Ryoho.* **29,** 2031–2036.
24. Sobrino, B. and Carracedo, A. (2005) SNP typing in forensic genetics: a review. *Methods Mol. Biol.* **297,** 107–126.
25. Hampe, J., Wollstein, A., Lu, T., et al. (2001) An integrated system for high throughput TaqMan based SNP genotyping. *Bioinformatics* **17,** 654–655.
26. Giles, J., Hardick, J., Yuenger, J., Dan, M., Reich, K., and Zenilman, J. (2004) Use of applied biosystems 7900HT sequence detection system and Taqman assay for detection of quinolone-resistant Neisseria gonorrhoeae. *J. Clin. Microbiol.* **42,** 3281–3283.
27. Borodina, T. A., Lehrach, H., and Soldatov, A. V. (2004) Ligation detection reaction-TaqMan procedure for single nucleotide polymorphism detection on genomic DNA. *Anal. Biochem.* **333,** 309–319.
28. Ahmadian, A., Gharizadeh, B., Gustafsson, A. C., et al. (2000) Single-nucleotide polymorphism analysis by pyrosequencing. *Anal. Biochem.* **280,** 103–110.
29. Odeberg, J., Holmberg, K., Eriksson, P., and Uhlen, M. (2002) Molecular haplotyping by pyrosequencing. *Biotechniques* **33,** 1104–1108.
30. Agaton, C., Unneberg, P., Sievertzon, M., et al. (2002) Gene expression analysis by signature pyrosequencing. *Gene* **289,** 31–39.
31. Holland, P. M., Abramson, R. D., Watson, R., and Gelfand, D. H. (1991) Detection of specific polymerase chain reaction product by utilizing the 5'–3' exonuclease activity of Thermus aquaticus DNA polymerase. *Proc. Natl. Acad. Sci. USA* **88,** 7276–7280.
32. Livak, K. J. (2003) SNP genotyping by the 5'-nuclease reaction. *Methods Mol. Biol.* **212,** 129–147.

33. McGuigan, F. E. and Ralston, S. H. (2002) Single nucleotide polymorphism detection: allelic discrimination using TaqMan. *Psychiatr. Genet.* **12,** 133–136.
34. Ranade, K., Chang, M. S., Ting, C. T., et al. (2001) High-throughput genotyping with single nucleotide polymorphisms. *Genome Res.* **11,** 1262–1268.
35. Livak, K. J. (1999) Allelic discrimination using fluorogenic probes and the 5' nuclease assay. *Genet Anal.* **14,** 143–149.

15

Genotyping Single-Nucleotide Polymorphisms by Matrix-Assisted Laser Desorption/Ionization Time-of-Flight-Based Mini-Sequencing

Xiyuan Sun and Baochuan Guo

Summary

Currently, there is a critical need to develop high-throughput, low-cost, and accurate methods for genotyping of single-nucleotide polymorphisms (SNPs). The matrix-assisted laser desorption/ionization time-of-flight (MALDI-TOF) mass spectrometrically based technique represents a new promising approach to SNP analysis. We have developed a new MALDI-TOF-based mini-sequencing assay, termed "VSET," for genotyping of SNPs. In this assay, specific fragments of genomic DNA containing the SNP site(s) are first amplified, followed by mini-sequencing in the presence of three ddNTPs and the fourth nucleotide in the deoxy form. In this way, the primer is extended by only one base from one allele, whereas it is typically extended by two bases from another allele. The products are then analyzed using MALDI-TOF mass spectrometry. The genotype of the SNP site is identified based on the number of nucleotides added.

Key Words: Genotyping; SNPs; MALDI-TOF; mini-sequencing; genetic variation.

1. Introduction

The most common polymorphisms in the human genome are single-nucleotide polymorphisms (SNPs). Once the site of an SNP is determined, the most important attribute of the SNP that requires being determined is its frequency in various populations and the correlation between its inheritance and any phenotypes such as a disease trait *(1)*. Several matrix-assisted laser desorption/ionization time-of-flight (MALDI-TOF) mass spectrometrically based mini-sequencing methods have been developed for genotyping of SNPs *(2)*. PINPOINT assay is promising as a result of its potential to identify multiple SNPs in a single tube *(3–5)*. In this assay, a primer is annealed to the targeted DNA immediately upstream of the SNP site and is extended by a single base in

From: *Methods in Molecular Medicine, Vol. 128: Cardiovascular Disease; Methods and Protocols; Volume 1*
Edited by: Q. Wang © Humana Press Inc., Totowa, NJ

the presence of all four ddNTPs. The base at the SNP site is identified by the mass added onto the primer. However, this method is limited by two problems. One problem is resolution, as the mass difference between nucleotides can be as little as 9 Da, and this renders it difficult to unambiguously identify the added nucleotide. The second problem is the salt effect, which renders it more difficult to accurately measure the peak masses as a result of the presence of Na^+, Mg^{2+}, and K^+ adducts.

PROBE is another promising mini-sequencing method in which the primer is extended in the presence three dNTPs and the fourth nucleotide in the dideoxy form *(6–8)*. In this way, the primer is extended by the addition of the ddNTP from one allele, while it is extended through the addition of dNTPs until the ddNTP is incorporated from another allele and the number of dNTPs added depends on the template sequence. However, this may create long extension products which can lead to several problems for multiplex genotyping. First, the long extension products may overlap with those produced from other SNP sites; second, the long extension products may not be detectable if extension is not efficient; and third, the presence of double charged and dimmer ions can be a problem since they may overlap with singly charged monomer ions.

Recently, we developed an alternative mini-sequencing method in which the primer is extended in the presence of three ddNTPs and the fourth nucleotide in the deoxy form *(9)*. In this way, the primer is extended by one of the ddNTPs from one allele, whereas it is normally extended by the addition of one dNTP, and then terminated by a ddNTP from another allele. Because this approach produces very short extension products, it is termed VSET (Very Short ExTension) assay. A VSET assay typically consists of four major steps: (1) PCR amplification of specific fragments of genomic DNA containing the SNP site(s); (2) mini-sequencing of PCR products; (3) purification of the mini-sequencing products; and (4) analysis of mini-sequencing products by MALDI-TOF. The genotype of the SNP site is identified based on the number of the new peaks and number of the nucleotides added (*see* **Fig. 1**). The main aspect of this method is that it can overcome the key problems associated with the other currently used methods. First, VSET greatly relaxes the stringent high-resolution and extensive desalting requirements that are essential to PIN-POINT. Second, VSET avoids the long extension problem associating with PROBE. In addition, this assay can be multiplexed to genotype multiple SNPs in a single tube reaction format (*see* **Note 1**).

2. Materials (*see* Note 2)

1. PCR DNA template: human genomic DNA extracted from blood, cultured cells, or tissues. The preferred template quantity is 10–100 ng.
2. Each of the PCR primers is synthesized according to the target SNP site. The preferred size of the PCR products is 100–150 bp in length.

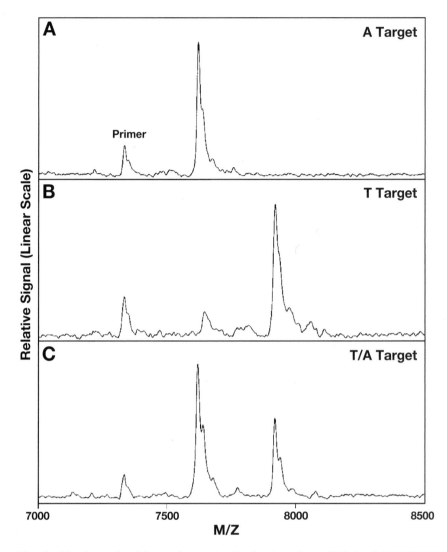

Fig. 1. Matrix-assisted laser desorption/ionization time-of-flight (MALDI-TOF) mass spectra of the primer extension products produced from A target or homozygote (**A**); T target or homozygote (**B**); and T/A target or heterozygote (**C**). (Reproduced from **ref. 9**, with permission from *Nucleic Acids Research*).

3. Mini-sequencing primer should be designed to anneal to the targeted sequence immediately upstream of the SNP site. Both strands of DNA can be targeted.
4. Shrimp alkaline phosphatase, Exonnuclease I, and ThermoSequenase can be obtained from Amersham Pharmacia Biotech. Taq DNA polymerases can be purchased from many sources.
5. 10 *M* Ammonium acetate.

6. 100 and 70% Ethanol.
7. 3-Hydropicolinic acid.
8. 50% Acetonitrile.
9. 0.1 *M* Ammonium citrate.
10. Pipets.
11. Centrifuge.
12. PCR thermal cycler.
13. MALDI-TOF mass spectrometry.

3. Methods (*see* Notes 3–5)

3.1. PCR Amplification

20 μL of the PCR reaction mixture includes 1X PCR reaction buffer, 0.2 μ*M* of each dNTP (dATP, dCTP, dGTP, dTTP), 2 m*M* of $MgCl_2$, 0.05 U/μL of Taq DNA polymerase, 0.1 μ*M* of each of forward and reverse PCR primers, and 10–100 ng of human genomic DNA. PCR is performed according to routine protocols and thermal cycling parameters.

3.2. Mini-Sequencing

1. Treat the PCR reaction products by adding 1 U of shrimp alkaline phosphatase and 1 U exonuclease I to the PCR reaction tube, followed by incubation at 37°C for 30 min, then 80°C for 10 min.
2. Add 5 μL of the treated PCR reaction products to 5 μL of the mini-sequencing mixture of 1X PCR buffer, 2 m*M* of $MgCl_2$, 1 μ*M* of mini-sequencing primer, 0.1 U/μL of ThermoSequenase, and 0.05 m*M* of each of the three ddNTPs and 0.05 m*M* of the dNTP. Primer extension is performed in 25–40 cycles.

3.3. Purification of Mini-Sequencing Products by Ethanol Precipitation

1. Add one-third volume of 10 *M* ammonium acetate solution to the mini-sequencing reaction tube (the final concentration of ammonium acetate is 2.5 *M*).
2. Add 4 vol of cooled 100% ethanol (ethanol final concentration of 80%), mix gently, and incubate it at –20°C for 30 min.
3. Centrifuge at 4°C for 20 min at 14,000*g*.
4. Discard the supernatant and wash one time by cooled 70% of ethanol.
5. Heat the tube at 70°C for 10 min to dry the DNA.
6. Add H_2O 5 μL to resuspend the DNA.

3.4. MALDI-TOF Analysis

1. 3-HPA matrix preparation: dissolve excessive amounts of 3-hydropicolinic acid (3-HPA) in 50% of acetonitrile and 0.1 *M* of ammonium citrate to freshly prepare the saturated 3-HPA matrix solution.
2. MALDI sample preparation: mix equal amounts of the purified mini-sequencing products with the 3-HPA matrix solution and deposit 0.5–1 μL this mixture onto a MALDI-TOF target. Let the sample dry in air.

3. MALDI-TOF mass spectrum acquisition: acquire mass spectra in a linear, negative ion, and delayed extraction mode. Fifteen or more shots are averaged to improve S/N. An example MALDI-TOF mass spectrum resulting from genotyping three individuals at the position of 1691(G/A) of Factor V is shown in **Fig. 1**.

4. Notes

1. This method can be used in multiplex genotyping of SNPs in a single tube, in which multiplex PCR is first performed to amplify the sequences containing the target SNP sites, followed by multiplex mini-sequencing to generate primer extension products.
2. All of the reagents should be of standard molecular biology purity grade. Use sterile distilled or deionized water.
3. Multiplex PCR is performed in two PCR rounds using chimeric primers that have both a hybridization segment and a constant segment *(10)*. In Round 1 of PCR, the hybridization segment hybridizes to the template to generate the specific sequences containing SNP sites and to attach the constant segments that do not hybridize with the original template, to the specific sequences. In Round 2 of PCR, the specific sequences produced from Round 1 and two primers containing only the sequence of the constant segments are used as template and primers, respectively.
4. Extension primers should be 15–30 bases in length. For multiplex VSET, it is important that the extension primers are designed to ensure that the primer and extension products do not overlap with each other. For example, we can use five sets (15, 18, 21, 24, and 27mers) of oligonucleotides as the extension primers for a 30-fold assay. The primers of different sizes are created with a 3' portion of the sequence complementary to the target and a 5' portion that is not complementary to the target. The 5' portion of the sequence serves as mass tag. In addition, six primers are created from each of the five sets and the average mass difference is about 50 Da among the six primers. This mass difference is sufficiently large to avoid the overlapping between the extended and unextended primers.
5. Desalting of mini-sequencing products can also be achieved by ion-exchange if the high resolution is not required. In this case, ion-exchange resins (in the form of H+) are first treated by 10 M NH_4Ac, followed by adding the resins to the mini-sequencing tube and incubation for overnight before analysis by MALDI-TOF.

References

1. Landegren, U., Nilsson, M., and Kwok P. Y. (1998) Reading Bits of Genetic Information: Methods for Single-Nucleotide Polymorphism Analysis. *Genome Res.* **8,** 769–776.
2. Guo, B. C. (1999) Mass spectrometry in DNA analysis. *Anal. Chem.* **71,** 333R–337R.
3. Roskey, M. T., Juhasz, P., Smirnov, I. P., Takach, E. J., Martin, S. A., and Haff, L. A. (1996) DNA sequencing by delayed extraction-matrix-assisted laser desorp-

tion/ionizaton time of flight mass spectrometry. *Proc. Natl. Acad. Sci. USA* **93,** 4724–4729.

4. Haff, L. A. and Smirnov, I. P. (1997) Single-nucleotide polymorphism identification assays using a thermostable DNA polymerase and delayed extraction MALDI-TOF mass spectrometry. *Genome Res.* **7,** 378–388.

5. Haff, L. A. and Smirnov, I. P. (1997) Multiplex genotyping of PCR products with MassTag-labeled primers. *Nucleic Acids Res.* **25,** 3749–3750.

6. Köster, H., Tang, K., Fu, D., et al. (1996) A strategy for rapid and efficient DNA sequencing by mass spectrometry. *Nat. Biotechnol.* **14,** 1123–1128.

7. Fu D. J., Tang K., Braun, A., et al. (1998) Sequencing exons 5 to 8 of the p53 gene by MALDI-TOF mass spectrometry. *Nat. Biotechnol.* **16,** 381–384.

8. Braun, A., Little, D. P., and Köster, H. (1997) Detecting CFTR gene mutations by using primer oligo base extension and mass spectrometry. *Clin. Chem.* **43,** 1151–1158.

9. Sun, X., Ding, H., Hung, K., and Guo, B. (2000) A new MALDI-TOF based minisequencing assay for genotyping of SNPS. *Nucleic Acids Res.* **28,** E68.

10. Wang, D. G., Fan, J., Siao, C., et al. (1998) Large-scale identification, mapping, and genotyping of single-nucleotide polymorphisms in the human genome. *Science* **280,** 1077–1082.

Index

A

Array comparative genomic
    hybridization,
    data analysis, 29
    genomic DNA label preparation,
        27–29
    hybridization, 28, 29
    materials, 24–26
    microarray construction, 26, 27,
        29
    principles, 23, 24, 29
    slide coating with aminosilane,
        26, 29
    washing, 28, 29
AVID, comparative genomics, 115

B–C

Berkeley PGA, *see* Programs for
    Genomic Applications
BLASTZ, comparative genomics,
    115, 116
Capillary electrophoresis, polymerase
    chain reaction amplification
    products, 131, 132
Cell fusion, *see* Somatic cell hybrids
Chromosome substitution strains
    (CSSs),
    applications, 166–168
    construction,
        crosses to substitute autosomes
            from donor strain, 161, 162
        genome scanning, 164, 165
        genotyping, 163
        homozygosing selected
            chromosome, 164
        host and donor strain selection,
            160, 161

mitochondria chromosome
    substitution from donor strain,
    162, 163
overview, 160
speed-consomics with marker-
    assisted selection, 163, 164
X chromosome substitution from
    donor strain, 162
Y chromosome substitution from
    donor strain, 162
historical perspective, 165, 166
quantitative trait loci,
    detection, 155, 157, 166
    mapping,
        congenic strain production,
            159, 160
        crosses, 157, 159
        dominance effect testing, 159
    resources, 168–170
Comparative genomic hybridization,
    see Array comparative
    genomic hybridization
Congenic strain, production with
    chromosome substitution
    strain, 159, 160
CSSs, *see* Chromosome substitution
    strains
Cytogenetic analysis, *see* Fluorescence
    in situ hybridization;
    Karyotyping

D

Denaturing high-performance liquid
    chromatography (dHPLC),
    long QT syndrome mutation
    detection, 183, 198, 199, 202,
    203